The Autism
Toilet Training
HANDBOOK

Essential Strategies for Home and School

MARY J. WROBEL

The Autism Toilet Training Handbook
Essential Strategies for Home and School

All marketing and publishing rights guaranteed to and reserved by:

FUTURE HORIZONS

(817) 277-0727

(817) 277-2270 (fax)

E-mail: info@fhautism.com

www.fhautism.com

ISBN: 9781957984087

Dedication

This book is dedicated to Eleanor, Wallace, Isla, and Cora. You are my inspiration and my heart.

Acknowledgments

Special thanks to Allison Rothamer for her suggestions, contributions, and editing of this manual. Thanks also to the many students, parents, and teachers who helped inspire the information in this booklet.

Contents

Contents

Contents

THE AUTISM TOILET TRAINING HANDBOOK

Introduction

Whether you have a child with autism or another disability, toilet training can often be a struggle and at times may seem to be an impossible achievement. But we know that being able to use a toilet independently and successfully is an important skill for everyone. Society expects children to, ideally, be toilet trained by the time they enter school, allowing them to fit in and function independently, like their peers.

Individuals who can't reach a level of toileting independence will need to depend on the assistance of adults and will often be segregated from other students in school, and later possibly segregated from others in society, perhaps for the rest of their lives. Not being able to independently use a toilet limits what a person can do and where they can go. It impacts their social acceptance and self-sufficiency, and further isolates them from their peers. If a person doesn't learn to use the toilet on their own, they will always be dependent on others to help them, and unfortunately, this makes those individuals much more vulnerable to molestation and sexual abuse. Learning to use a toilet isn't just convenient and cost-saving; it is important for a person's safety, independence, and social-emotional health.

If a child or older individual is physically capable of using the toilet, they should be able to be toilet trained, regardless of their cognition, level of anxiety, sensory sensitivities, or language capabilities. It is my hope that this manual will help parents and educators with the arduous task of teaching children with ASD the very important skill of using the toilet.

Autism & Toilet Training

Toilet Training is Difficult Whether a Child has a Disability or Not

Teaching a child to use a toilet is difficult even if the child doesn't have a disability. Adding a disability to the task of toilet training can make it monumentally challenging. Many professionals believe that children with autism spectrum disorder (ASD) are more challenging to toilet train than any other population due to their rigidity, dislike of change, sensory issues, and innate anxieties. Their various language and communication challenges are also a major factor to understanding, following through on tasks, and expressing their questions and feelings during the process of toilet training. Those who have attempted to toilet train a child (or adult) with ASD by following popular toilet training methods often very quickly find that they are as ineffective as they are stressful, for all involved. And because autism is a spectrum disorder, this means each individual can be very different from others with ASD, and approaches for teaching them will vary from one individual to another. In other words, that means there is no approach to toilet training that will work with all individuals with ASD.

Toilet training for an ASD individual is not quick or easy. Toileting plans that offer quick results can often backfire and cause a child to have more fear and be more resistant to the process. Becoming an independent toilet user is a long process, even for neurotypical children, and setbacks and accidents are to be expected. It's not only a learning process for the child, but for the parents as well, who often dread the time when they need to introduce the concept of using the toilet versus wearing diapers. It can be a difficult and stressful transition involving a lot of time, effort, and patience.

Readiness Often Isn't the Issue

It's widely believed that a child needs to be physically, mentally, and emotionally ready before the process of toilet training can begin. We often hear parents and teachers comment that a child who is still in diapers just "isn't ready" to use the toilet. Parents and teachers will look for signs from the child that indicate the child is ready to comprehend use of the toilet, as well as being physically and emotionally mature enough to begin the toilet training process. For the neurotypical child, that period usually begins between the ages of 2 and 3.

Parents of autistic children may therefore also try to introduce toileting when their child is of a typical toilet training age (usually by the time their child is 3 or 4 years old), and they hope or assume their child is ready. But what frequently happens is that the attempt fails and parents completely stop the toilet training and go back to using diapers, because the attempt was too stressful. The parents may then assume that their child simply isn't ready to transition to the toilet and may decide to wait for a later time when they think their child will show signs of readiness. Unfortunately, a child with ASD may never actually feel that readiness. Furthermore, every time the toileting process fails and as the child grows older, the harder the toilet training process becomes. The truth is that a child with autism may never really feel "ready" to be toilet trained, and the longer parents wait for that "sign of readiness," the harder the process will likely become.

While it is true that all individuals with autism are different, it's a very common trait among autistic individuals to have a difficult time with change. We know that people with autism (including children) hate sudden changes to routines. Any necessary change to a routine often requires a slow introduction, consistency, and time before that change is accepted and can be established as a new routine. If wearing diapers is all a child has ever known, the very concept of going from wearing diapers to eliminating into a toilet is a massive (and terrifying) change to everything a child is used to and understands regarding elimination.

The failed attempts to teach kids to use the toilet often inadvertently ends up teaching them to fight even harder against that change. When a child with autism fights against using the toilet, and the parents give up, the child comes away with the understanding that by resisting, they can continue using the diapers that they feel comfortable with and don't want to give up. Therefore, each time parents attempt to start the toilet training over again, it becomes harder and harder, and often with stronger and stronger resistance from their child. This resistance often consists of screaming, crying, refusal to cooperate, and possibly destruction and aggression.

How Schools Succeed When Parents Fail

It's understandable then why parents, incredibly stressed out by the entire ordeal, will give up and revert to using diapers. Because at that point, the diapers are the easier and more convenient option, and creating a peaceful home environment is naturally a higher priority to parents than having their child use a toilet. Eventually the task of toilet training is often left up to the child's classroom teacher and school staff. The school is often very successful, even after parents have failed countless times. This is especially true in a self-contained classroom that teaches toileting skills to diaper-wearing students. It's not because the child is finally "ready" for toileting, but because the school establishes a specific toileting routine, which they implement consistently every day, often supported by visual aids and Social Stories™. Schools tend to have this rigid structure built into their daily routine, whereas a home environment is typically much less structured.

Scheduled toilet breaks at school may be set for every hour, two hours, or longer as the child learns the routine for using the toilet. These scheduled breaks train the child to use the toilet, whether they need to go or not, and help them to be successful.

The student may initially fight the toileting routine, but because the routine is part of the school schedule and is always consistent, eventually the student accepts it and participates. Not only does the student's individual toileting ritual become part of the routine at school, but it also soon becomes the rule for toileting everywhere.

Unlike parents, teachers can remove emotional investment in the toileting process. Teachers can be patient with the process and take the toileting procedures slowly, gearing the expectations to each individual child. Students are typically put on a consistent toileting schedule, which they learn to anticipate each day. When toileting becomes a part of the school routine, with established rules specific to that routine, it's simply a matter of time before acceptance and success follow.

A school also has the advantage of making and using materials that help with learning toileting skills, such as picture schedules, visual supports, and Social Stories™. These teaching aids help to establish the individual, broken-down steps of toileting and teach the necessary vocabulary related to using the toilet. Visual aids help to teach children the behavior that is expected of them regarding all aspects of toileting. Additionally, they can address unexpected problems such as, "What if there's no toilet paper?" or "What if I have a mess in my underwear?" By addressing specific toileting problems, teachers can use visual aids and discussion to help students learn to problem-solve. Therefore, many kids with autism become successful using the toilet at school before they do at home.

The Autism Toilet Training Handbook

If your child is in school, you will want to coordinate with the school staff to get some of those supports to help you with toileting at home. That way, there is consistency in all locations and situations. The more consistency there is with toileting across a variety of locations, the more successful the toilet-training process will be.

TIPS AND STRATEGIES TO REMEMBER:

- Think of the unique characteristics of your child which may help or hinder toileting.
- Plan the toileting process with your child's strengths in mind. What do they like? What are they good at?
- Your child may never feel "ready" to use the toilet. Fear of change is a powerful influence.
- Failed attempts to toilet train can lead to more resistance.
- How is the school addressing toilet training? What is working for them?
- Coordinate toileting plans with school.
- Replicate supports used at school for home.

Laying the Groundwork for Successful Toileting

When to Begin the Toileting Process

Since we know that many ASD students may never feel ready or motivated to use the toilet on their own, when should toilet training begin? There is often disagreement as to when to start the process, because again, very young children aren't physically, emotionally, or mentally able to use the toilet or potty chair successfully and make the transition from diapers to toilet.

When considering the best time to begin the toileting process, instead of thinking in terms of complete and successful skill acquisition, we should think instead about simply establishing routines and laying the groundwork for an easy toileting transition.

What does that mean exactly? If we think in terms of a child with ASD who has only ever known wearing and eliminating in diapers, hates change, and is perhaps fearful of using the toilet, it makes sense to begin the toileting process sooner rather than later. This might mean starting as early as eighteen months of age by introducing the potty chair as part of the bathroom routine.

Let me clarify by saying, you don't want to begin toilet training at eighteen months of age. Instead, you want to simply introduce the concept of sitting on the potty chair, without any expectation of using the potty chair. Sitting briefly on the potty chair just becomes added to the bathroom routine, perhaps before or after taking a bath, or as part of your child's morning or evening routine in the bathroom. The potty chair then never becomes something to be feared or refused, and it doesn't ever pose a sudden and drastic change to the child's day. It is simply one more addition to the bathroom schedule, and something familiar and expected.

Starting the toileting process at eighteen months might not be an option. We are now able to diagnose autism at earlier and earlier ages, but unfortunately, most children with autism still aren't diagnosed until age 2, 3, or older. It is understandable that after receiving a diagnosis of autism, parents are often overwhelmed, and the last thing they will be thinking about is toilet training. But toilet training shouldn't be overwhelming, at least not initially. Think about using Social Stories™ and visual supports to help your child prepare for and anticipate these changes. Small steps toward introducing the toileting routine to your child, even if your child is already three or older, is a way to lay the groundwork for happy and successful toileting down the road.

Start Diapering in the Bathroom

Most children reach a point when they know when they will have a bowel movement and will often find a quiet, secluded area of the home to do their business while wearing a diaper. If your child can anticipate needing to defecate and even asks for a diaper to "poop," put on their diaper in the bathroom and indicate to the child that pooping needs to happen in the bathroom, even if they are wearing a diaper. Allow them the privacy of doing their business in the bathroom if they want to be alone. This helps them understand that bathrooms are private places and toileting with or without a diaper needs to happen in a bathroom.

Another way to establish the idea that all toileting belongs in the bathroom is to begin by doing all diaper changes in the bathroom. This might be inconvenient and possibly uncomfortable for the parent and child, but remember, the purpose of this new change is to establish the rules that all toileting, including changing diapers, belongs in the bathroom. Changing diapers in the bathroom allows you and your child to put solid waste in the toilet and flush it. It also gives you the opportunity to talk about why we use the toilet, and it establishes the idea that pee and poo belong in the toilet. Again, don't expect too much from your child at this point. You simply want to establish a happy bathroom routine with little or no fear. Taking small steps is key.

TIPS AND STRATEGIES TO REMEMBER:

- Start early, or as early as possible, to prepare for a smooth transition.
- Take it slowly and don't put expectations on your child.
- Create new bathroom routines, using the potty chair or toilet.
- Discuss toilet use and how mommy and daddy, etc. use the toilet.
- Help your child feel comfortable near a potty chair or toilet.
- Use Social Stories™, support stories, and visual supports to help prepare your child for the changes to come.
- If your child asks for a diaper to do their business, have them wear the diaper and eliminate while they are in the bathroom.
- Diaper changes should start to take place in the bathroom once you introduce the concept of using the toilet/potty chair.

Getting Started

Begin with a Plan

Once you have decided to truly begin toilet training, you need to generate a plan with your family. This needs to be a plan you can stick with and not quit when it becomes difficult, and it's very likely that it will become difficult. To generate a plan, parents/caregivers need to write out their plan with step-by-step procedures. Included in those procedures should be how you, parents and caregivers, plan to respond to refusals and meltdowns. Additionally, you need to anticipate setbacks. Setbacks and failures will happen, but that doesn't mean you quit the plan. Adjusting for setbacks, but continuing with the toileting plan, is the goal.

Toileting is a Time Commitment

The idea that toileting can be accepted and mastered in a day will not work for kids with ASD or other disabilities. In fact, that approach shouldn't even be attempted. Forcing toilet training on a child with ASD will likely cause more anxiety and refusal behaviors and will probably stall any further toilet training for quite a while. Not only will the process take time, but there is a daily commitment as well. The ideal toilet training process will take things slowly, making only small changes at a time and allowing those changes to become thoroughly accepted and mastered before continuing forward and introducing any additional steps. This reduces stress and decreases the likelihood of errors and setbacks. Break toileting down into many small steps and make forward progress, small step by small step. This way, if you hit a particularly rough spot in training, you can take a step or two back without it unraveling too much of their progress.

Issues to Consider

Before beginning the process of a toileting plan, you will need to address any anxiety and sensory issues, which your child may have. Anxiety and sensory issues aren't unique to the ASD population, but these issues tend to be more intense for individuals with autism and can be very impactful to toilet training.

Language and communication are also an issue. Many children with autism struggle with comprehension of oral language and typically have difficulty expressing themselves effectively. If a child doesn't have an effective communication system, which is appropriate to their needs, then attempting to toilet train could be disastrous. Such a child will likely use behavior to communicate their confusion, fear, anger, and anxiety. Behaviors such as meltdowns, aggression, destruction, and refusals can immediately stop any toileting progress.

TIPS AND STRATEGIES TO REMEMBER:

- Generate a toileting plan with your family (and anyone else who may be involved with the toileting process) before beginning actual toilet training.
- The plan should have small, step-by-step procedures and address any problems that may occur along the way.
- Commit to the Plan! You need a plan you can stick with, no matter what happens. So, make sure your plan is realistic and modifiable,
- Toilet training can take time and feel very stressful. Take it slowly.
- Before starting a toileting plan, address any possible anxiety, sensory processing issues and language/communication difficulties your child may have.

Language & Communication

Addressing Language/Communication Needs

Just because a child has some verbal language and can sometimes express themselves verbally doesn't mean they will comprehend what you tell them or verbally express themselves well all the time. The definition of ASD includes deficits in language, communication, and social skills, and most people with autism struggle with these language/communication/social deficits their entire lives. Individuals with ASD, especially children, tend to be visually strong and depend on visual supports to help them comprehend verbal language. We can't assume they will understand what we say when we explain the steps to using a toilet or following through on a bathroom routine, even if we use simple words and directions.

Before beginning any toilet training, a child needs a means to communicate their feelings, as well as wants and needs. They also need a way to understand what an adult is explaining and directing them to do. This is where a communication system, visual supports, and Social Stories™ become necessary.

Effective Communication Systems

A communication system is only appropriate if the person it's designed for can understand it and use it with some independence and communicative intent. Usually, simple is best. Parents and school staff often want to use more complex communication devices, which may be difficult for a child to navigate and use. Also, communication folders or books with too many pictures and categories can make it hard for a child to find and quickly communicate what they want/need. If a child is not yet proficient at using a more complex communication system, scale it back or use multiple, simpler boards or screens with less pictures.

If a child has a communication system that works for them, use that in the bathroom when explaining a task and encouraging them to respond. It may also be helpful to create a new communication board or folder with specific pictures and terminology related to toileting. When creating a board or folder for the bathroom, remember to use the pictures your child is familiar with (such as Boardmaker or another picture system). Above all, it's important that your child understand the pictures when using any visual support. When using any picture system, point to the picture of what you are saying while explaining or asking questions. Then allow the child to respond by using the pictures as well.

It's important to use a communication system that your child will understand and can use with minimal help. There are many systems to choose from, such as communication boards and folders with pictures and words, alphabet boards for spelling out words, iPads, tablets, and specific voice output devices. Almost all of these systems use pictures, either abstract, line-drawn pictures, or photos. Once a child understands pictures as they relate to verbal language and can navigate a picture system or device to find the picture they need to communicate, they will be ready for more detailed or complex picture systems or devices. When a child understands pictures and can use a picture system, they will be able to understand a variety of visual supports that can be incorporated into the toilet training process.

Picture Exchange Communication System

If your child doesn't have any effective means to communicate, consider having them learn to use the Picture Exchange Communication System (PECS). This is a great first communication system and particularly essential for children who are non-verbal and don't have a consistent and appropriate way to communicate. Check with a Speech-Language Pathologist or check online to learn how to use this communication system. PECS is a very effective, almost no-fail system for teaching a young child how to communicate their wants and needs, especially if they have never yet learned to use a picture system to communicate.

Communication Boards and Folders

Communication boards and folders are simple, take up little space, are easy to use, and often are topic-specific. Because of this they are ideal for using in the bathroom, especially if they are laminated. Ask school staff or private therapists to help you create and laminate any communication boards you may need for home. If your child's school is already using specific boards and folders at school, have them duplicate those for home use, as needed.

Behavior is Communication

Remember language and communication is essential when attempting to teach the various tasks necessary for toilet training. If a child doesn't have an appropriate means to understand the language an adult is using and respond to that language effectively, they will resort to using behavior to communicate. And often that behavior can be inappropriate and volatile, especially if the child is upset, anxious, or angry. Always try to get a child to use pictures or other more appropriate means to communicate their feelings, confusion, and questions.

TIPS AND STRATEGIES TO REMEMBER:

- Comprehending verbal language and communicating verbally are often difficult for a child with ASD.
- Every child should have an effective communication system they can use independently.
- ASD individuals tend to be visually strong and need visual supports to comprehend verbal information.
- Use pictures or a picture system a child understands and is familiar with.
- Use communication boards and folders in the bathroom. They're simple and easy to use and can be topic-specific.
- Behavior is communication. Children with ASD who don't have a way to appropriately communicate will use behavior (e.g., screaming, crying, throwing things, covering ears, self-abuse, aggression) to communicate.

Addressing Anxiety

Autism and Anxiety

Most professionals would agree that anxiety is a major part of the autism experience. Signs of anxiety can be seen at a young age and will often become more intense, diverse, and overwhelming as children get older. Anxiety impacts the lives of individuals with ASD in various ways. It can cause ASD kids to be afraid, have panic attacks, and exhibit task refusals and lack of cooperation. ASD individuals may demonstrate shutdowns, meltdowns, aggression, and regression. Toilet training, not surprisingly, constitutes a huge change and is very stressful and anxiety-inducing. Even kids who don't have autism often have major anxieties about using the toilet.

Anxiety is almost certain to factor in the task of toileting. This is especially true for kids who begin the toilet-training process at an older age. As children with ASD grow older, they establish more rigid routines and have less tolerance for change. Consequently, anxieties begin to manifest and complicate any change and the learning of new tasks, including toilet training.

Regardless of at what age a child with ASD is learning to use the toilet, we can't ignore the potential of anxiety and should always anticipate its influence. Kids with autism experience anxiety more intensely and often more frequently than other children. Parents and staff who know that a child exhibits anxieties need to expect and recognize anxiety triggers.

Possible Anxiety Triggers for Children with ASD

Kids with autism aren't all the same, and each will experience anxiety in their own unique way. Likewise, every child may have anxiety triggers that are unique to them. Some common anxiety triggers for ASD individuals include:

- Changes or disruptions in routine
- Changes in the environment
- Not knowing what to expect
- Unfamiliar people and settings
- Fear of a situation
- Loud unexpected noises
- Overstimulating environments
- Overwhelming sensory stimuli
- Unpredictable occurrences
- Transitioning from one activity to another

Strategies and Incentives to Tackle Anxiety

If you know what triggers a child or student, prepare them for what will happen and help them with strategies and incentives. For example:

1. Explain calmly what will happen in detail. A Social Story™ is an excellent way to prepare someone for something anxiety-producing. Don't wait until the last minute to tell them what will happen or try to trick them into a task that you know will produce anxiety. In the case of toileting, tell them specifically what they will be doing and how long it will last.

   Social Stories™ are best used when a child is calm and in a good mood—this is when the information is best absorbed. When a child is in the throes of anxiety, it's not a good time to try to reason with them about what is expected of them. Once a child is melting down emotionally, they aren't in a state of mind where they can rationalize, so these attempts will usually only aggravate the meltdown. In this situation, it's usually best to simply be a calming presence and help the child calm themselves in whatever way best suits them. But when your child is in a good mood and nothing stressful is being asked of them—that's a great time to go over a toileting Social Story™ with them!

2. Remind them of incentives: show them what they will earn by taking part in the toileting task. Make sure the incentives are something they really want.

3. Give them strategies for overcoming their anxieties, but also know when something is so overwhelming that you must stop the task or activity.

4. Provide a bin of sensory toys and allow them to take a sensory break or use sensory toys while on the toilet.

5. Give them an escape plan. If they clearly can't handle the situation, don't push them to the point of a complete breakdown. Give them a phrase or action they can use that indicates they need a break.

6. Always, always encourage them and let them know that they are doing their best to comply. Tell them that you know they are trying.

Often, young children with autism don't recognize when they are feeling anxious. They may not know that the bad feelings they are experiencing, and the accompanying behaviors, are due to anxiety. It is difficult even for neurotypical children to recognize that what they are feeling is anxiety. On top of which, they need to recognize the cause, have the ability to communicate this to others, or know how to appropriately help themselves feel better. This is something even many adults struggle with. With this in mind, we should be extra understanding for autistic youth. As adults, we may need to make note of the signs of a child's anxiety and possibly explain to the child that what is happening to them is due to their anxiety.

Possible Signs of Anxiety:

- Sudden, intense fear
- Heart beats quickly
- Feeling sweaty and hot
- Feeling nauseous, dizzy, and confused
- Feeling claustrophobic
- Exhibiting obsessive behavior
- A sudden desire to run away or escape
- A sudden feeling of being frozen and unable to do anything
- Exhibiting excessive self-stim behaviors
- An intense need to keep people at a distance, even aggressing toward people when they get too close

It should also be noted that for many neurodivergent (ASD or ADHD) individuals, anxiety can induce a very calm appearance, with very little facial expression or bodily movement. In these individuals, anxiety produces physical behavior that presents more like a body going into shock. Many people may assume their child is not anxious because their physical features don't appear to present as being anxious, when in fact, under the surface, their entire self is practically numb from the weight of enormous anxiety.

Strategies to Help a Child Calm Down

If you know your child has anxieties, find strategies that will help your child calm down and feel less anxious. Some children when anxious want to be comforted by a caregiver, while others need space. Giving a child what they need for comfort looks different for all children. Let each child determine which strategies are most helpful for them. Not all strategies help all children, and your observations, as well as the child's input, are important for determining which strategies work and which don't. The following are examples of strategies to reduce or stop a child's feeling of anxiety:

1. Have your child breathe deeply with eyes closed, perhaps with their head between their knees while adult counts slowly to 10.
2. Take a break. Allow your child to leave the room or the task for a while and do something that isn't stressful. Give them a choice of break activities.
3. Incorporate movement, such as heavy sensory activities or going for a walk. A change of scenery, plus movement, helps ease anxiety.
4. Turn on music that your child likes. Allow your child to pick happy, enjoyable music or calm, relaxing music.
5. Do a relaxing activity, something you know your child likes to do.

6. Do something with your child that makes them laugh or smile. Laughter eases anxiety.
7. Provide a happy distraction, something that gets their attention and pulls them away from anxious thoughts.
8. Give your child a favorite comfort toy, such as a stuffed animal that they can cuddle with.
9. Give your child a sensory toy or a deep sensory massage to help them relax.
10. Finally, assure your child that soon anxious feelings will go away and they'll feel calm and happy again.

Everyone feels anxious sometimes. Explain to your child that anxious feelings might be with us for a while, maybe a short time, or maybe a bit longer—but eventually we all become calm again, and they will be calm again, too. Remember that anxiety is a big hurdle when it comes to toilet-training a child. So, while you begin creating a toileting plan for your child, anticipate and plan for episodes of anxiety. Once children can reduce or overcome their anxieties, they will be more successful with toileting.

TIPS AND STRATEGIES TO REMEMBER:

- Anxiety is a part of autism and typically becomes more problematic as a child grows older. Toileting is often a major source of anxiety for kids with ASD.
- Be aware of the anxiety triggers which can cause a child to go into anxiety mode (see possible triggers in this chapter) and have a plan in place for when anxiety occurs.
- Help a child understand the feeling of being anxious and give them strategies to help them become calm (see strategies in this chapter)
- Have a bin of sensory toys on hand to allow them a sensory break if they need it and allow the child to choose the available sensory toys in their bin.
- Give them a means to request a break if a situation becomes too overwhelming.
- Remind them of incentives/rewards to help them stay on-task and move through their anxieties.
- Use support stories or Social Stories™ to address their fears, prepare for any anxieties, and help them manage those situations.
- Remind them that they will feel calm again and reward them for trying their best.

Addressing Sensory Sensitivities & Aversions

Autism and Sensory Sensitivities

Many individuals with autism have sensory sensitivities and aversions which may contribute to an inability to use the toilet. Sensory sensitivities have to do with processing sensory information. Our nervous systems take in sensory information in each environment by means of our senses. How we process and manage that sensory information determines whether we can handle it or have specific sensitivities to it. Every child with autism is different when it comes to sensory sensitivities. Some children can barely stand such things as bright lights, loud noises, specific textures and certain smells and tastes, while other children seem to need and are distracted by more intense sensory stimuli. It helps to know exactly what those sensitivities and responses are before implementing a toileting plan. Sensory issues can vary AND involve more than one sense. Not all sensory issues are tactile—you could be dealing with auditory sensitivities, sensitivities to smell (olfactory), or sensitivity to things like temperature or pain.

Children with autism can be hypersensitive to certain input (which means they are easily overwhelmed by sensory stimulation and need less of it), and they can also be hypo- or under-sensitive to certain input (where that sensory input isn't enough, and they seek either more or higher intensities of it). To add further complication to a child's sensory processing, a child with ASD can be hyper-sensitive to some input in specific environments and hypo-reactive to other sensory input within the same environments. For this reason, it is important to determine how your child reacts to a variety of stimuli in the bathroom before beginning the process of toilet training. They may be hyper-sensitive to some sensory input as well as hypo-reactive to other stimuli all in the same bathroom environment. You need to find out what is impacting your child's sensory processing and address it before expecting toileting success.

Common Hyper-Sensitivity Responses:

- Covering their ears in the presence of noise, or in anticipation of noise
- Closing eyes or not looking at certain lighting or bright colors
- Screaming or crying in the presence of a smell/taste/sight/sound/touch that is overwhelming
- Complaining or irritability about something overstimulating

- Running from anything overstimulating
- Excessive self-stimulation (stimming): rocking, arm flapping, etc. to cope with overwhelming stimuli
- Aggression toward others when overwhelmed by sensory information or in anticipation of unwelcome sensory

Signs of Hyper-Sensitivities in the Bathroom:

- Not wanting to sit on a hard or cold toilet seat
- Afraid of toilet water splashing on their bare bottom
- Upset by sounds: toilet flushing, water running, air hand dryers, exhaust fans, etc.
- Overwhelmed by smells, either pleasant (air fresheners/ soaps) or unpleasant
- Wanting the lights and/or exhaust fans off
- Not wanting to use soap or wash hands, an aversion to brushing teeth and showering, and sensitivity to too-hot or too-cold water

Children who are hypo-reactive to certain sensory information may crave or need stronger sensory stimulation. Parents and staff may assume that individuals with ASD who are hypo-reactive would do better with toileting, but that's not necessarily true. Individuals with hypo-reactive sensitivities can be very easily distracted by sensory stimuli, which can also lead to problematic behavior in the bathroom. Like hypersensitive individuals, those with hypo- or weak sensory perception will also self-stim. However, in their case, it is to INCREASE their sensory input.

Common Hypo-Sensitivity Responses:

- Ignoring certain sounds, including people talking to them
- Liking loud, echoing sounds
- Focusing on bright, intense, or blinking lights
- Seeking more intense stimulation of sight/sound/taste/smell/touch, including harsher fabrics, and needing to feel hard or course textures on their skin
- Self-stimulation (stimming) to increase sensory input

Signs of Hypo-Sensitivities in the Bathroom:

- Repeatedly flushing the toilet
- Repeatedly washing hands or desiring very hot/cold water or high water pressure
- Flicking lights off and on
- Staring at lights or ceiling fans
- Distracted by listening to the exhaust fan or other sounds in the bathroom
- Licking surfaces
- Touching and smelling urine and feces

Questions to Think About Regarding a Child's Sensitivities in the Bathroom

Ask yourself these questions about your child before implementing your toileting plan:

- Is the toilet seat too cold or hard for my child's sensitivities? Is it too soft?
- Is the toilet opening too exposing for their bottom?
- Is the sound of the flushing toilet auditorily overloading? Do they like to flush repeatedly?
- Is the smell of the toilet overwhelming? Are there some other smells (like an air freshener) that are simply too much?
- Is your child anxious and therefore in need of sensory stimulation (squeeze ball, small blanket, toy, etc.) to calm them while in the bathroom?
- Does your child not like the feel of toilet paper? Or of a particular toilet paper? Do they like to use excessive amounts of toilet paper?
- Are the acoustics in the bathroom too loud or disturbing? Are they distracted by loud noises?
- Are they distracted by sensory stimuli in the bathroom and have difficulty staying on task?
- Is there something else in the bathroom causing a sensory issue, such as fluorescent lights? (Fluorescent lights are a

very common complaint among autistic individuals.) Or do they spend too much time staring at the lights?

- How can I make the bathroom environment a pleasant one for my child without overloading their senses?
- How can I keep my child on task in the bathroom when they are distracted by sensory stimuli?

Handling Sensory Issues in the Bathroom

If you discover a sensory sensitivity with your child, do what you can to address those sensitivities or aversions. If necessary, change the toilet seat or the toilet paper. Neutralize the smells in the bathroom or perhaps infuse a scent that's pleasing to your child. Change the lighting to a softer light. Have favorite music playing in the bathroom if that's what they want.

If you can't change an overwhelming sensitivity to something, or if it's necessary that they to learn to eventually handle it, begin by gradually increasing the amount of time they are exposed to whatever is overloading their senses. By gradually increasing their tolerance for certain sensitivities, they will not only overcome intolerances to their home bathroom, but will learn to tolerate other bathrooms as well.

Self-stimming is often a coping mechanism for handling anxiety, as well as for handling overwhelming sensory input. Have a small bin of sensory toys/objects nearby in case they need it for coping with sensory overload or underload. Use visual supports and Social Stories™ to help them prepare for possible sensitivities, reactions, or aversions. Do what you need to do to make the toileting experience a pleasant one.

If your child is seeking or distracted by sensory stimuli, find ways to minimize those distractions. Reward on-task behaviors with desired sensory stimuli. If they have a hard time transitioning from a desired sensory stimulation, implement an If-Then reward system (example: *If* you sit on the toilet for a few seconds, *then* you can turn on the exhaust fan) and allow them to choose a sensory toy or activity after they complete a toileting task. Reward them for *not* doing gross or unhygienic behaviors, such as licking surfaces or touching/smelling feces.

Remember, sensory overload and sensitivities are real and can affect your child in several ways. Occupational therapists have several approaches for dealing with sensory processing disorders and can help with strategies for handling hyper and hypo responses to sensory information. If you need additional strategies for dealing with your child's sensory issues, contact OTs at school or in private practice to help with sensory regulation. Almost everyone with autism has a sensory processing disorder of some kind, and often they have more than one. Don't ignore these sensitivities, as they have a direct effect on a child's behavior and capabilities.

A Case Study

Consider the case of Lucy, a nine-year-old child with ASD who failed repeatedly to successfully use the toilet. Lucy had good awareness and excellent control of her urinations and bowel movements. She was able to withhold her eliminations until she was wearing a diaper, and only then would she allow herself to eliminate.

Lucy had serious sensory issues and anxieties, which included loud noises and tactile sensitivities, such as hard surfaces and cold water. She couldn't stand the feeling of defecating in the toilet. But when she had the security of wearing a diaper, she was comfortable enough to eliminate. She also refused to sit on an open toilet because it felt too exposing for her. Even though she was able to occasionally pee in a potty chair, she had an ongoing problem with sitting on the toilet and exposing her naked bottom. When she was put on an open toilet, she would scream and fight her parents and teachers.

Lucy was too big to use a potty chair anymore. Furthermore, using a potty chair at school wasn't an option. It became clear that due to Lucy's sensitivities and aversions with the toilet, we needed to begin the toilet training with her wearing a diaper.

We began by using visual supports and a Social Story™ to help Lucy understand her new toileting plan at home. Soft lighting and minimized noise helped to establish a pleasant environment in the bathroom. With her parents' help and calm reassurance, Lucy would sit on the open toilet seat while wearing her diaper. She was directed to eliminate into her diaper while sitting on the toilet. She was allowed a selection of sensory toys and books to help her relax. After she was able and comfortable doing that, her parents would cut out the center of her diaper so that her bottom was partially exposed and some of her elimination would go into the toilet. Lucy was comfortable doing this because she still had the security of wearing her diaper, as well as a soft toilet seat insert, which helped her feel less exposed. Bit by bit, more of her diaper was removed, until all her elimination was going into the toilet. Soon she was able to make the decision to sit on the toilet seat with just the soft insert and no diaper. It was important to let her decide when to stop wearing her diapers, a decision she made when she was finally comfortable enough to give them up. Eventually, Lucy was able to transition to a hard toilet seat and could successfully use the regular bathrooms at school.

When dealing with sensitivities and aversions, it's important to take it slowly to allow your child to get used to new and uncomfortable feelings and sensations. Using a toilet feels very different than eliminating in a diaper. This is a huge change for someone with autism to handle comfortably.

TIPS AND STRATEGIES TO REMEMBER:

- If you know your child has sensory processing problems and sensitivities, determine if those sensitivities present themselves in the bathroom and while toileting.
- A child can be hypersensitive to some sensory input and hypo-reactive to others. It's not uncommon for a child with sensory processing issues to be hyper- and hypo-reactive to a variety of sensory stimuli (see examples of hyper and hypo sensitivities/reactions in the bathroom in this chapter).
- Ask yourself questions regarding the bathroom environment that may be impacting your child's sensory response (see questions above).
- Change what you can in the bathroom to minimize sensory sensitivities (e.g., neutralize odors, change lights, add favorite music)

- If you can't change something in a bathroom or they need to manage their sensitivities in other bathroom environments (such as a school bathroom), gradually increase their exposure and tolerance to it and prepare them to handle their sensory sensitivities. Continue to encourage them and reward them for handling sensory stimuli.
- If a child seeks and is distracted by sensory stimuli, find ways to minimize those distractions and reward them for staying focused on the toileting task (use an IF ___ THEN reward system and reward them with more sensory stimuli after they complete the toileting task). Reward them for *not* doing any unhygienic behaviors, such as licking surfaces.
- Seek the professional advice of Occupational Therapists (OTs) if you need more strategies for handling sensory processing issues.

Creating a Toileting Plan

Start with What Your Child Can Do and Is Comfortable Doing

If your child screams at the sight of the toilet, you wouldn't start your plan with having your child sit on it. You might first begin with simply looking inside the toilet, learning about the parts of the toilet, flushing the toilet, and just generally feeling comfortable around the toilet. If you need to begin from farther away because your child doesn't even want to go near the toilet, then start by getting your child comfortable being just inside the bathroom, but not too close to the toilet. Figure out your child's threshold of comfort, and work on getting closer from there. If your child has anxiety about defecating even in their diaper, then start there—reward pooping in the diaper, and work on thoroughly alleviating that anxiety before trying to get them to use the toilet. Start wherever your child needs to start, rather than where you think the toilet-training should be started.

Consider Toilet Training with a Potty Chair

Potty chairs are smaller and low to the ground, making them easy to use. Sometimes kids are afraid that they will fall into the toilet, but that won't happen with a potty chair. Furthermore, potty chairs don't flush, so they aren't as noisy or scary. A potty chair might not be possible if you are toilet training an older child or adult. In that case, use a toilet insert in a standard toilet. A toilet insert will make a standard toilet seat more comfortable and less intimidating and allow for less exposure on the toilet.

Allow Your Child to Choose Their Potty Chair or Toilet Seat Insert

Your child will be more invested in using a toilet insert or potty chair if they can choose which one to use. There are lots of potty chairs, many with themes and pretty designs. Some potty chairs have music, cheering, and even artificial flushing sounds. Your child might like all the bells and whistles in a potty chair, or none of that. For this reason, it's important to allow your child to choose their own potty chair. Likewise, toilet seat inserts can come in various colors, designs, and sizes. Many inserts are padded, making them soft and more comfortable to use. It's also important that a child decide on which to use—a toilet insert or the potty chair. However, larger children might not be afforded a choice between potty chair and toilet. Bigger and older children should use the toilet, possibly with an insert, versus the smaller, less accommodating potty chair.

Think in Terms of Small Steps

Think about all the steps involved with using a toilet or potty chair. Break down each step into smaller ones. Think in terms of what you know about your child and what they can accomplish. We might think of an instruction such as "wash your hands" as being simple enough, but to a child in the process of learning their bathroom routine, this needs to be broken down into a list of specific tasks in a specific order: turn on faucet, wet hands, put soap on hands, rub/lather hands for a count of ___ seconds, rinse soap under faucet, turn off faucet, dry hands.

Set Schedules and Routines

Insert the toilet or potty chair into your child's daily routine, even if it's just talking about it at first. Eventually you will want your child to do something with the potty chair/toilet, whether it is calmly touching it or sitting on it briefly, perhaps wearing a diaper. After a bath, before they are dressed, let them sit on the potty chair or toilet while they are waiting to be dressed. There are many ways to insert the potty/toilet into your child's daily bathroom routine. Make a visual schedule that shows all the steps to your child's bathroom routine, including a step involving the toilet/potty chair.

Take It Slowly

This should be a given. Toilet training is a long process. Successful toilet training can take several months and even years. Don't get excited or impatient and rush the steps of your plan, and don't jump ahead if you think your child is ready to skip a few steps. Skipping steps can cause anxiety and setbacks, and you'll want to avoid those, if possible.

Work with School

If your child is attending school, talk with school staff about the bathroom routines they incorporate and what is working for them. Try to be consistent between home and school. Discuss your child's anxieties and sensory sensitivities with school and make them aware of triggers and behaviors associated with those anxieties and sensitivities. Let school staff know any successful strategies you use at home for calming your child down. Calming-down strategies may need to differ from home and school, but making school staff aware of what is done at home will help them develop similar plans at school. Finally, ask school staff for help in creating visual supports and Social Stories™. It's important that school and home follow a consistent plan and routine together. Continuity is very important for toilet training success.

Commit to the Plan

Even if along the way you need to make changes and adjustments, don't abandon the plan altogether. Remind yourself that setbacks will happen, and take a step or two back to what your child can comfortably do. Think about why there is a setback. What is the roadblock? Has anything changed? Has a recent event upset your child? Is your child confused about what is expected of them? Do you need more visual supports or strategies to handle any anxiety or other problems? Setbacks will always happen, but if we don't figure out why a setback occurred, we won't be able to fix it and move forward.

Parents/Caregivers Need to Stay Motivated

Toilet training is a long, hard process with plenty of roadblocks. It's hard to stick to a plan if you are feeling defeated or you don't think progress is being made. Often parents long to take the easy way out and just go back to diapers, etc. It's important that adults who are involved in the process of toileting a child with ASD learn to stay motivated despite any problems. Parents and other family members need to find ways to reward themselves when their child makes progress. Remember that YOU are also working hard to help your child learn to use the toilet! Ways to stay motivated:

1. Adults should reward themselves with a night out, a special activity, or even a glass of champagne when their child makes progress.

2. Small progress is hard to see. Chart your child's progress to see how far they've come. This will help keep you motivated.

3. Have regular family meetings and pep talks to discuss progress with those involved in the toilet training, and brainstorm solutions to any problems which may come up.

4. Plan for adult rewards (what you want to do) when your child achieves a major goal. This could be a plan with or without your child.

What's important is not to give up on the plan despite any setbacks or large problems.

Use Support Stories and Visual Supports

These supports will help your child understand the expectations, learn the appropriate steps to using the toilet, predict what will happen next, manage their emotions and anxieties, and learn to problem solve. Ask the school to help with this. The school staff can make supports for you to use at home. Details about visual supports and Support Stories are in later chapters in this book. Please refer to those chapters when you want to create or get examples of those supports.

TIPS AND STRATEGIES TO REMEMBER:

- Start at the step your child is comfortable doing. That may be just looking at the toilet and flushing it. Adults don't decide which step to begin the toileting plan. A child's comfort and capability decide where you start.
- Consider starting with a potty chair-they are easier to use and less intimidating for your child.
- If a child is too big for a potty chair use a toilet insert on the toilet seat.
- Kids should choose the potty chair they want to use. They come in a variety of colors, designs, and accessories.
- Insert potty time, even briefly, into your child's bathroom routine. Establishing a routine with the potty allows for a smooth transition when you begin toilet training in earnest.
- Be consistent between home and school. Establish an ongoing means of communication about toileting between home and school.
- Expect setbacks and adjust or make changes, but don't abandon the plan.
- Parents and caregivers need to find ways to stay motivated and not give up.
- Don't forget to use Social Stories™ and visual supports, especially when there are setbacks.

Rewards & Incentives

Think carefully about the rewards and incentives you plan to use when potty training your child, because they may be the only motivators to get your child to use the toilet. Kids with autism aren't usually motivated by social acceptance and social rules. They don't always care about being like mommy/daddy or big brother/sister or any of their classmates who use the toilet. Social pressure will not motivate them. In fact, your child could be the only one in pre-school or kindergarten who still wears a diaper and that will be perfectly fine with them. It is more important to your child to be comfortable and do what they routinely do, rather than face a fearful change. Remember, if wearing a diaper is all they have ever known, then making the change to using a toilet will be huge and scary for them.

The key to getting your child with autism to voluntarily (and happily) use the toilet is to find the incentives and rewards that will motivate them. Each child is different, and most parents have a good idea what their children wants the most. Before beginning a toileting plan, parents need to follow these important strategies:

When and How to Reward

- **Reward small steps and each small goal accomplished.** For example, if you have a goal of your child overcoming their fear and just simply sitting on the toilet for a few seconds, then reward them for doing that.
- **Reward immediately.** Don't wait until your child has achieved five stars/stickers before they can receive a prize. Most kids with autism won't understand the concept of delayed reward or the idea that they need to achieve a set number of stars before they get a prize. If the reward is too far away or seems too difficult to attain, the child will lose interest.
- **Keep rewards small and simple.** Don't reward your child with big, expensive gifts each time they accomplish a goal. If your child wants a big, expensive gift, save that for the end. It can be the final prize for accomplishing toileting.
- **Give a choice of rewards.** Allow your child to choose the reward from a small selection of choices. Don't give the same reward each time, unless that is what your child chooses. Variety is important to help keep your child motivated, which means you may need to occasionally switch the choices of rewards to something new and exciting.
- **As the goals become harder, think of creative ways to reward:**

MYSTERY PRIZES

Your child might like the idea of getting a special
surprise, such as a small, wrapped present they can
open or choosing something unseen from a box of prizes.
Many children are particularly motivated by a mystery prize.
Plastic easter eggs are an easy way to hide small prizes.

UNEXPECTED REWARDS

Switching up or varying prizes can keep kids from becoming
bored. If you always reward with stickers, for example, your
child might lose interest in stickers.

BREAK BIG PRIZES INTO SMALLER REWARDS

If your child likes certain toy sets, giving them an entire toy
set as a reward would be too excessive for completing small
steps, but withholding it until total success may make it seem
unattainable. Instead, you can have your child select a toy
set, and you can open it and remove and wrap up individual
pieces, and reward with those individual mystery pieces. This
keeps your reward highly motivating, exciting, and attainable,
AND it allows kids to see and enjoy their own progress. Lego,
puzzles, and magnetic tile toys are great if your child enjoys
building things, for example.

USE PICTURE CARDS

Bigger prizes can include treasured activities or snacks, and
while you may not be able to immediately reward these, you

can use something like a picture card to represent this prize. If your child has earned themselves a trip to their favorite fast-food location or a treasured snack at the store, you can't immediately give that reward, but it's very important to give your child something physical to represent that. ASD kids in general tend to be very visual learners, and handing them a picture to represent a delayed reward will be much more effective than simply telling a child "You earned a trip to ____!"

- **Keep praise matter-of-fact and not over-the-top.** Too much excitement and praise can be overwhelming for your child. The same is true if they can't do the step they are expected to accomplish. Don't show huge disappointment! Be matter-of-fact if they fail and say, "That's okay, maybe next time you can do it." Always be encouraging.
- **Don't exhibit anger or negative reactions, and don't ever punish for setbacks!** This goes without saying. Negativity of any kind can cause your child to shut down and refuse to participate.

Examples of Small Rewards:
- A small treat (cookie, cracker, chip, candy)
- A sticker (if that's something they like)

- Small, cheap toys that you know your child will like
- Puzzle pieces, if they like puzzles, until the puzzle is complete
- Pieces of any other type of toy set, like Magnatiles
- Watching a favorite movie or show on TV
- A new book
- A favorite activity such as cooking, bubbles, jumping on a trampoline

Examples of Bigger Rewards:
- Trip to McDonald's or another favorite restaurant
- Special toy
- A purchased movie (DVD)
- A trip to a special store, park, or playground
- A train ride
- A trip to the zoo
- A trip to the beach, lake, or pool

TIPS AND STRATEGIES TO REMEMBER:

- Strong motivation, not social pressure, will encourage your child to participate in toileting.
- Find a variety of very motivating incentives for your child.
- Remember to reward immediately.
- Keep most rewards small and save big rewards for big achievements.
- Be creative with your rewarding and give reward choices (see above).
- Keep praise matter-of-fact (nothing over-the-top).
- Never punish for setbacks or noncompliance. Stay away from negativity.

Implementing the Plan

Preparing to Implement

Meet as a team, parents and school staff (if your child is in school), before beginning your child's toileting plan. Determine what your child can do already at home and at school, then compile a list of small goals for your child to complete. Keep the goals small so you can ensure success for your child. You don't want to overwhelm them with too many steps at once or goals that are too hard for them to achieve. By keeping your goals small, your child can make steady progress toward the goal of completing toilet training.

Determine a start date for the toilet training, but avoid starting right before or after a holiday, birthday, or significant event, as that will add stress and likely overwhelm your child, as well as all involved in the toileting. Parents often like to begin toilet training in the summer, when there is less stress and it is a more relaxed time of year for everyone. If, however, parents want to coordinate with school, begin the home toileting program on a weekend, hopefully a long weekend. Clear off all weekend events and begin the home toileting on a Friday or Saturday. Start by reading one or two Social Stories™ and introducing visual supports, as well as the toileting schedule. Have everything prepared and ready before you begin. Schools should consider beginning a toileting plan at the start of the school year when the teacher is establishing the classroom schedule.

Remember not to rush it, and avoid jumping over goals when you think your child can handle it. Sometimes a child can handle initial steps without a problem, but there will be goals that are too much for them, and they may refuse to cooperate. When you reach a roadblock, instead of shutting down the whole toileting process, take a step back to a goal that you know they can accomplish and feel comfortable doing before moving forward again.

Remember: you are creating a new routine for your child, a routine that they are not yet comfortable doing. There will be resistance and possible meltdowns, but stick with the plan, remain calm, and take it slowly. During the entire toilet training and small-step goals, always explain to your child what you are doing and what they need to do. Don't pretend or try to trick them. Always be honest and reassuring. And when they are afraid or have difficulty, don't overreact. Remind them that they are doing a good job, and no matter what they do, it will be okay.

At some point, with much preparation, you may need to ditch the diapers and forge ahead with the toileting plan. Permanently removing diapers, at least for day-training, will be a big but necessary step. When the diapers are gone, be prepared for setbacks and toileting accidents, and be forgiving of both. Despite all the preparations, when the diapers disappear, it will be a dramatic and difficult change for your child.

Visual Supports

Before, during, and even after successfully toilet training your child, use visual supports. Visual supports can help your child understand what they need to do, as well as showing the steps involved in the process.

Sometimes when talking about what your child needs to do, a picture not only helps them understand the task, but also helps alleviate any fears. Adults often try to verbally explain a task or situation to an ASD child without realizing that most of what they say is not understood, or not auditorily processed and remembered. Kids with ASD are typically visual learners and therefore need visuals to help them understand, as well as to communicate their feelings and responses.

The visual supports should be pictures, photos, or written steps that your child will understand. If your child already uses a communication system that uses line drawings, such as Boardmaker pictures, then use that same system of pictures when making visual supports.

If you need to use photos, look online. There are a variety of online sites that provide photos to help teach kids with disabilities. You may find that using a combination of photos, line drawings, and words are the best options to help your child really understand. Almost any type of visual will work if your child can look at a picture and understand what it means when it's coupled with a verbal response.

Use visual supports to show step-by-step instructions for your child to do. Visual supports posted in the bathroom can serve as a reminder of what they need to do with the order of the tasks involved. If your child forgets a step or becomes confused, they can look at the visual reminders in the bathroom to help them confidently finish their toileting task.

If the idea of using visual supports is too overwhelming or difficult for you as a parent, contact the school or your child's private therapists for ideas and help in creating any needed materials. Visual supports and reminders allow your child to be independent and private in the bathroom, which is the end goal for successful toileting.

EXAMPLES OF VISUAL SUPPORTS YOU MAY NEED:

- **A numbered and illustrated step-by-step list** of what they need to do when using the toilet, posted in the bathroom *these lists can be broken down into specific tasks with separate lists for the toilet, toilet paper use, adjusting clothing, and using the sink.
- **An illustrated daily schedule**, which shows all the times for scheduled toileting throughout the child's day (home and school).
- **Illustrated, personalized Social Stories™** using photos or abstract drawings.

- **An Illustrated "It's Almost Time for the Toilet" sign** with a picture of the toilet, which can be used to transition a child from an activity they are doing to using the toilet.
- **A visual timer**, which doesn't make noise but instead counts down the time with a visual strip. This can be used to transition to bathroom time or as a timer when they're on the toilet.
- **An illustrated reminder** of any step they may forget posted by the toilet.
- **A First-Then folder**, which shows the pictured task: "First" on one side of the folder and the reward for doing the task, "Then" on the other side of the folder. The tasks and rewards should be able to be switched for different ones. Consider using Velcro, sticky tack, or even tape to adhere the task (First) and (Then) reward pictures to the folder.
- **An illustrated list of incentives and rewards** that they can earn when using the toilet.
- **A small, illustrated sign of praise**, (e.g., Good Job! You Did It! Try Your Best! You Are Amazing!) posted in the bathroom for encouragement.
- **An illustrated, personalized song** about using the toilet that they can sing (or that someone can sing to them). This is a great way to calm them, distract them, or help them relax.
- **Picture reminder cards** that mom/dad/caregiver are there to help whenever anything feels overwhelming. *They can also use those cards to indicate they need help.*
- **A "Something Has Changed" card** that shows a picture of anything involving a *change* to the bathroom routine or bathroom

environment. It's always important to let a child know about *any* changes to their bathroom routine, including scheduling, no matter how small.

- **A break card** in case a task becomes too overwhelming and they need a break.
- **A list of illustrated strategies** to help them calm down. If they get upset or anxious, a list of pictured strategies from which they can choose will help them calm down, including sensory objects they can ask for, which aren't readily available in the bathroom.
- **An illustrated communication folder** specifically for the bathroom, which will express their feelings, communicate their wants and needs, and answer their questions.
- **A feelings folder** with *I Feel:* on one side and *Because:* on the other. Have a variety of pictured feelings on the *I Feel* side, such as sad, upset, anxious, nervous, confused, happy, okay, distracted, mad, and uncomfortable. On the *Because* side, show a variety of pictured reasons for the feeling your child chooses, such as: "I'm afraid," "it's too loud," "the toilet hurts me," "it hurts to poop," "the lights bother me," and "I did a good job." It helps adults to know how a child is feeling and why during setbacks and problems. Boardmaker (Mayer-Johnson) has pictures for all the above feelings and reasons.
- **Photos of them using the toilet and following through on toileting tasks**. *Sometimes it helps for them to see themselves doing a good job performing those tasks to understand how they look doing the toileting routine. When they see photos of*

themselves during the toileting process (sitting on the toilet, washing hands, etc.) it gives them pride for a job well done and encourages acceptance of that task.

These visual supports can be posted in the bathroom, or used just prior to, or in some cases after using the toilet. Don't just post these visual supports; go over all of them with your child (or student) so that you know the child understands what the supports mean and how to use them. For many with autism, visual supports are vital for helping them understand, communicate with others, and remember what they need to do.

Steps Toward Achievement

The following is an example of goals/objectives you can use with your child during the toilet-training process. Begin at a level that you know your child can already do successfully. Remember to reward them when they achieve a goal.

- They can look at and touch the toilet without fear.
- They can lift the toilet lid and look inside.
- They can flush the toilet without fear (with lid closed).
- They can flush the toilet with lid open and watch the water go down.
- They can sit on the closed toilet seat fully clothed.
- They can sit on the open toilet seat fully clothed.
- They can sit on an open toilet seat in diaper (or underwear).

- They can dump solid waste (feces) from a diaper or underwear into the toilet.
- They can flush solid waste and watch it go down.
- They can sit on an open toilet seat with bare bottom for a second or more.
- They can sit on an open toilet seat with bare bottom for 30 seconds or more.
- They can comfortably sit on an open toilet seat with bare bottom for a minute or more.
- They can comfortably sit on the toilet three or more times a day for a minute or more.
- They initiate sitting on the toilet when it is suggested.
- They are able to sit on more than one toilet (e.g., school, home, other toilet) comfortably.
- They can comfortably sit on the toilet and occasionally (accidentally) urinate.
- They can use toilet paper with assistance.
- They can perform appropriate toileting routine (sit on toilet, use toilet paper and drop in toilet, pull up pants, flush toilet, and wash hands) with assistance.
- They can perform appropriate toileting routine independently with visual aids or verbal cues.
- They can wear underpants instead of diapers during the day.
- They can tell you when they "need to pee."
- They can urinate in the toilet 1–3 times a day.

- They can indicate when they need to "poop."
- They can sit on the toilet and attempt to "poop."
- They can defecate in the toilet occasionally.
- They can defecate in the toilet 1–3 times a day.
- They can wipe their bottom with toilet paper after a bowel movement with physical assistance.
- They can wipe their bottom until clean without assistance.
- They can eliminate in the toilet and follow all the steps of the toileting routine independently.
- They are able to know when they need to use the toilet and can do so without being told.
- They can use the toilet consistently and successfully with few or no accidents.
- They can remain dry at night.
- They can get up at night to use the toilet if they need to.

These are only examples of goals to use with your child or student. Each child is different, and you may need to become creative or more specific with the goals you choose. If your child has a sensory processing disorder or sensory sensitivities, for example, you may need to include goals that address that. If your child has cognitive or physical limitations, your goals may need to change to make the toileting process easier.

It's important that you adhere to a step-by-step progression using the samples of steps provided. In the progression of toileting skills, children are often more comfortable and able to urinate in a toilet before defecating. Nighttime accidents are often the norm for many kids before they have the bladder control and the ability to wake up when they need to go.

Creating a Schedule and Routine for Home

The following is an example of a schedule you might want to use. Remember, the plan you devise for your child must be individualized to fit the needs of your own child. Keep your child hydrated with plenty of water, especially during the day. This is important for kids with autism, since they tend to be dehydrated anyway. Drinking plenty of water will help your child be able to urinate when the time comes.

- **First thing in the morning:** child enters bathroom after waking up. Diaper is removed and disposed of properly. Child sits on potty chair/toilet. Parent asks child if they need to "pee." If not, child gets off potty chair, washes hands, and continues their usual bathroom routine. If the child eliminates in the toilet/potty chair, they receive a small reward.
- **Before leaving for school:** child enters the bathroom, diaper or underwear is removed, and child sits on potty chair. After a minute or two, if child doesn't eliminate, they pull up pants (adult puts on diaper), wash hands, and continue bathroom routine (e.g., brushing teeth). If they eliminate in the potty chair, they receive a small reward.
- **Upon arriving home from school:** child immediately enters the bathroom, pulls down pants, and sits on the toilet/potty

chair. They follow the toileting routine and are rewarded if they eliminate in the toilet.

- **Before dinner:** child enters bathroom, sits on toilet/potty chair, and follows the toileting routine, with the final step of washing hands before leaving the bathroom. Again, the child is rewarded if they eliminate in the toilet.

- **After dinner:** if your child typically eliminates after dinner, go to the bathroom and have them sit on the toilet/potty chair. As always, help your child through the bathroom routine, and reward if they eliminate in the toilet or potty chair.

- **Before bed:** child sits on the toilet/potty chair as part of the bedtime bathroom routine with the same expectations and toileting routine. Again, they are rewarded if they eliminate in the toilet.

Don't force your child to sit **TOO LONG** on the toilet/potty chair. You want to keep the amount of time on the toilet short, hopefully productive, and, above all, pleasant. If, however, your child indicates that they need more time on the toilet, allow them to sit longer. Children with ASD often have a poor concept of time. Some respond well to setting a timer (visual timers are best) to allow them to know how long they need to sit on the toilet or stay in the bathroom. Keep them entertained while they sit. Use a short song as a measure of time and sing it while they are sitting on the toilet. Read them a short book while they are on the toilet. Choose an activity they will enjoy (such as playing a game on a tablet) to help them relax and remain seated on the toilet.

If, at the end of the time period for sitting on the toilet, your child hasn't done anything, be reassuring and matter-of-fact, and help them go through the rest of the toileting routine: use toilet paper, flush toilet, pull up underpants and pants, wash hands with soap and water, and finally, dry hands on a towel before leaving the bathroom. If they are successful and eliminate in the toilet, give brief praise and reward them immediately, then continue with the toileting routine.

TIPS AND STRATEGIES TO REMEMBER:

■ Determine a start date not near any important event.

■ Make or compile a list of small goals for your child to complete and rewards after each success. Refer to your goal list frequently to know what was completed and what's next (see "Steps Toward Achievement" in this chapter).

■ Make a variety of visual supports and stories to have on hand in the bathroom to use before, during, and after the toilet-training process (see all the suggestions listed above). Make sure the child understands what each support means and how to use it.

■ Create a toileting schedule and routine for home, beginning first thing in the morning and ending before bed.

■ Despite any setbacks, resistance, or meltdowns on the part of the child, adults should remain calm and encouraging.

■ Don't force a child to sit too long on a toilet/potty chair. Make the sitting time on a toilet/potty chair as pleasurable for the child as possible.

■ Getting rid of the diapers will be a big change, and when the diapers are gone for good, prepare for setbacks, accidents, and possible meltdowns.

Charting Progress

Why Should You Chart?

If your child has a consistent schedule for meal/snack times, rest times, and active times, then they will likely have an elimination pattern that you can predict and plan around. This is important when remembering that autistic children don't always transition well from one activity in one area, to a different activity in a different area. This is especially true when you attempt a transition from an enjoyable activity to one that isn't. For example, if you know your child tends to need to use a toilet around 4 PM every day, you don't want to let them start watching a favorite show at 3:45, because that would be something that would be difficult for them to transition away from. Where possible, you want to schedule toilet breaks BEFORE those highly enjoyable activities. Children will come to expect "first toilet, then TV" or "first toilet, then snack," etc. That enjoyable activity can then serve as an additional motivator. Charting your child's toileting activity can help you get a good idea of how best to schedule their toilet breaks within the day.

Charting their child's toileting progress not only helps parents see how many times their child is successful and when the child is most successful, but also indicates where the setbacks or problems are. Charting gives a parent or teacher much clearer information regarding the entire toileting process with all the contributing factors. The best way to chart might be to have the date or time on the far-left side of your chart, with various charting categories across the top toward the right.

THINGS TO CONSIDER WHEN CHARTING:

- Time of day
- Child's mood: calm, sad, upset, happy, tired
- Sensitivities exhibited by child
- Motivator used
- Who assisted child in the bathroom
- Activity prior to toileting: playing, sleeping, outside, eating
- Cooperative or uncooperative behavior
- Elimination (if any)—urine or fecal
- Follow-through on toilet routine (toilet paper, flushing, pants up, wash hands)

Sample Chart

Date:

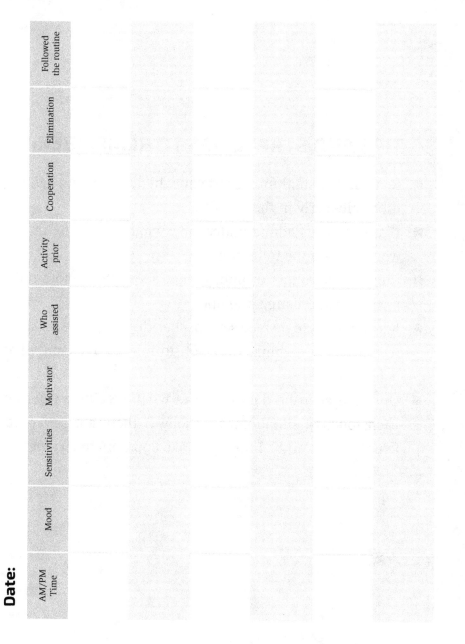

AM/PM Time	Mood	Sensitivities	Motivator	Who assisted	Activity prior	Cooperation	Elimination	Followed the routine

TIPS AND STRATEGIES TO REMEMBER:

- Remember to faithfully chart your child's toileting attempts, especially early in the process.
- Charting helps adults understand what is working or not working with the toilet training.
- Charting gives lots of information about the factors influencing each toileting attempt.
- It's important to include several charting categories, besides whether they eliminated or not, to fully understand what is happening.
- Once the charting data indicates what is going on during each toileting situation, especially if there are any problems, parents and adults can make appropriate changes.

Older Children & Toileting

What to Expect

Children five years and older who are involved in repeat toilet training or are being toilet trained for the first time have their own set of obstacles. Remember that past failures will influence future success. If your child has always used tantrums and aggression to avoid using the toilet, you will need to power through those behaviors with calm determination. Remember, too, that an older child with ASD is likely to exhibit more anxieties, which will add to their resistive behaviors. Many of these children already know what is expected of them with regards to using the toilet. And consequently, they may already have extreme anxiety about using the toilet before you even begin the process of toilet training. It's especially important to prepare your child with Social Stories™ and visual supports to help them understand what's expected of them and address their emotions and behaviors.

You may need to take it slow and start small. You may even need to start from scratch, with an emphasis on making the toileting experience as pleasant as possible. Spend a lot of time calmly talking about toilet use. Using Social Stories™ and visual supports, explain to them what you are doing, as well as what they will be doing. Address their fears and assure them that you will be there to help them.

If your child acts out and becomes aggressive during the toileting process, take a step back, if necessary. Establish rules about aggression and remind them that it's okay to get angry and upset, but it's not okay to hurt others or damage anything. Affirm their fears and anger but explain calmly that they still need to try. Let them know that you realize this is new and difficult for them, but you will be there to help with everything and soon they will be successful. Remind them, too, about rewards they will get when they do a good job. Always try to be positive and encouraging. Don't ever use threats or punishment to get them to cooperate.

Establishing New Routines

Probably the hardest task with an older child is establishing new toileting and bathroom routines. This will be hard because for several years they have become used to routines that don't involve using the toilet. They are comfortable with the routines they have had for those many years and will be especially resistant to change. Instead of changing their routines entirely, find ways to incorporate additions. They will be more willing to accept additions to their routines if they can keep the routines they know and like.

1. Make sure your child has a way of communicating their fears, anxieties, and upsets, especially if they are non-verbal or limitedly verbal. Always allow your child or student to use their method of communication whenever you are working on toilet training.

2. Work closely with school staff and use the same or similar plan at home. Find out what is working well at school regarding toileting and do that at home. As always, use visual supports and stories to help your child understand, accept, and cooperate with all the toileting steps.

3. Establish a highly motivating reward system. Incentives will be especially important to help them accept the new changes.

4. If your child is urinating and defecating at regular, predictable times, getting them on the toilet when you know they are likely to be ready to eliminate will help with toileting success. Remember that setbacks will happen, but it's your job as a parent to stick with the plan, no matter what, and not give up.

TIPS AND STRATEGIES TO REMEMBER:

- Past failures will influence future attempts at toilet training.
- Make sure your child has a way to communicate and use visual supports and stories they will understand.
- Once you decide to toilet train your child, don't give up!
- Expect difficult behavior and more anxiety, but power through it calmly and be reassuring. Have a list of strategies to manage behavior and anxiety.
- Be sure to have highly motivating incentives.
- Be prepared to re-introduce toilet training all over again, and implement a new, different routine around the times when they are more likely to eliminate.

Tackling Problems Associated with Toilet Training

Withholding

What is *withholding*?

When anyone refuses to defecate or urinate, medical problems ensue. Withholding urine and/or feces can cause any number of problems, including urinary tract infections, kidney and bladder infections, severe constipation, intestinal blockage, massive bowel impaction, and damage to the colon. Furthermore, to prevent the need to pee, a person may stop drinking or may drink very little, which causes dehydration, dizziness, and fainting. When children have a pattern of withholding, regardless of the reasons, the consequences are serious. Whether you are a child or an adult, withholding urine and feces causes physical problems, some of which may be long-lasting.

Withholding bowel movements, also known as paradoxical diarrhea, isn't uncommon among children ages two to four years old and usually correlates with toilet training. It can occur if a child has had a painful episode of constipation or as the result of fear of eliminating in the toilet. In the case of children with ASD, it can also result from a sensory processing disorder. Often kids with ASD who have sensory processing issues don't want to poop because they don't like how it feels. Sensory processing issues plus fear of elimination can cause children with ASD to withhold bowel movements.

Withholding can cause an individual to have an impacted bowel, and the longer a person goes without moving their bowels, the more painful and traumatic that elimination will become. Surprisingly, when a person's bowel is impacted, they appear to exhibit diarrhea. The diarrhea is a result of liquid waste escaping around the solid, impacted mass in the person's bowel. This liquid is called paradoxical diarrhea, but it is not actual diarrhea and shouldn't be treated as such. Because of this paradoxical diarrhea, parents can be fooled into thinking their child doesn't have constipation because of withholding. If the severe constipation and withholding continues, the problem can become much worse before it is correctly identified and eventually resolved.

If your child is withholding and refusing to defecate, this can become serious and may result in the need for medical intervention and possible hospitalization. Kids can go several days without defecating, but that is not healthy and can cause long-term problems. Ideally, people, including children, defecate two to four times a day, and this is what you want your child to be doing.

Children who have a pattern of withholding will eventually develop long-term bowel problems. It may develop into a vicious cycle of constipation, which would require medication and enemas to correct. If you suspect your child is withholding bowel movements and possibly urine to avoid using the toilet, you need to stop your toilet plan and make immediate changes. Since we know that withholding is serious with potential dire consequences, it is necessary at this point to evaluate the reason your child is withholding. You will also need to discuss your concerns with a doctor. If your child is attending school, contact the classroom teacher and school nurse to alert them to the situation. Find out if your child is withholding at school. Sometimes students with ASD don't like using the large, communal school bathrooms. They may refuse to use the school bathroom or other bathrooms because of sensory issues, dislike of the bathroom, or even bullying by others in the bathroom. Whatever the reason, it's always important to find out why a child is refusing to use a bathroom before attempting to address any withholding.

REASONS A CHILD MAY BE WITHHOLDING:

- Fear of sitting on the open toilet. This could be about falling in or feeling too exposed and vulnerable with a naked bottom on the toilet.
- Fear of losing a part of themselves into the toilet. They don't understand that poop is waste, not a piece of their body.
- Anxiety about using the toilet and not being able to use a diaper.

- Anxiety and fear about being splashed with toilet water while sitting on the toilet.
- Anxiety and fear about having to use different toilets and bathrooms.
- Sensory issues specific to the toileting experience in a particular location, such as sensitivities to sound, sights, smells, hearing, and touch.
- Dislike of any change.
- Fear due to potential bullying in a bathroom.
- Anxiety about using a different toilet than their "preferred" toilet.

Withholding is not just a problem for children learning to use the toilet. It can also develop with children and adults who are already successful and independent using the toilet. Preventing oneself from urinating and defecating is typically a choice made for one reason or another, and determining the reason behind someone's withholding behavior is vital. Withholding can happen at any age and for a variety of reasons, some of which may seem untypical or unreasonable. The following is an example of withholding that doesn't occur because of learning to use the toilet.

Withholding Case Study

A smart, articulate young woman with ASD told me that when she was in high school, she never used the bathrooms at school. She was comfortable using a variety of bathrooms and had been using toilets on her own for many years. Despite that, on her first day of high school when she attempted to use the bathroom, a group of girls in there bullied her and threatened her if she ever used a bathroom at school again. The young woman with ASD was frightened and took those threats seriously and therefore never used the bathroom at school during her four years attending high school. Instead of telling anyone about the bullying, she endeavored to solve the problem herself by refusing to eat or drink anything all day while at school. She thought if she didn't eat or drink, she wouldn't need to use the bathroom. During her long hours at school, she often felt faint, and she developed frequent bladder and urinary tract infections, as well as severe constipation. Her reason for withholding may seem outrageous or ridiculous to us, but to this girl with autism, it was the only solution she could think of. And because of threats by the bullying girls in the bathroom, she was afraid to tell her parents or school staff.

As this example shows, withholding for any reason can be a problem for someone, including older individuals with ASD and anyone who may already be proficient in independent toilet use. Withholding at school or other locations outside of the home is not uncommon for children with autism. Even if a child is successful and independent using a toilet, problems such as constipation and urinary tract infections, which don't have an obvious indication (such as poor diet or hydration) should alert parents and staff to determine what is causing those problems.

Constipation

Constipation is one of the most common bowel problems among individuals with ASD. The problem with constipation is that the longer fecal matter remains inside the bowel, the harder it gets. And the harder it gets, the more painful it becomes to pass. Constipation, also a symptom of withholding, can severely disrupt the function of a person's gastrointestinal tract. Constant smelly gas is often a sign of constipation; however, several additional signs can also indicate constipation.

SYMPTOMS OF CONSTIPATION:

1. Loss of appetite. Most people who are severely constipated often lose their appetite, as it becomes too painful or uncomfortable to eat.
2. Fewer than three solid bowel movements a week, often very large stools which may clog the toilet.
3. Paradoxical diarrhea instead of solid poops.
4. Abdominal pain.
5. Small, hard ball-like poops.
6. Anal pain and some bleeding when passing a bowel movement.
7. Extreme straining when trying to defecate.
8. Walking with stiff legs, sitting and standing in such a way as to indicate discomfort, in an effort to withhold bowel movements.

Correcting a child's constipation can be scary and traumatic for the child, especially if enemas and hospitalization are involved. Enemas are effective but typically uncomfortable and intrusive. Enemas are typically safe, but if administered incorrectly or repeatedly, they can cause tissue damage to the rectum and colon and possible bowel perforation. Other side effects of frequent enema use are infections, electrolyte imbalances, and occasional bloating and cramping. Laxatives can help soften stools and allow for easier bowel movements, but long-term use of laxatives is typically not recommended for young children. It can also cause problems with their gastro-intestinal systems. Laxatives might temporarily eliminate constipation, but once a person stops taking the laxatives the constipation will likely return, perhaps worse than before.

FACTORS CONTRIBUTING TO CONSTIPATION:

- Low-fiber diet and inadequate fluids
- Withholding bowel movements because the child insists that poop can only go in a diaper, not in a toilet
- Lack of interoceptive awareness, which gives a person the recognition and urge to poop
- Food allergies and sensitivities
- Various anxieties about using the toilet

Treating Constipation:

Things to try according to Maureen Bennie, *Constipation, Withholding and Overflow: A Deeper Dive into Bowel Problems for Individuals with ASD*, blog, 9/8/20:

1. Help your child relax their muscles by blowing bubbles or blowing into a whistle toy while sitting on the toilet.

2. Increasing fluid intake is very important! Have water readily available all over the house, anywhere your child may be. Use their preferred style of water bottles or cups, and regularly encourage water-drinking. For dental health, water is strongly recommended over other (especially sugary) beverages.

   Juices/milks/sodas are beverages that contain sugars, so they are best served with a meal or as a snack, while water should be the #1 beverage encouraged for regular hydration throughout the day. This way the teeth aren't frequently being coated in liquid sugars throughout the day.

3. Limit processed foods and increase high-fiber foods. Many autistic children are not as fond of fruits and vegetables due to the unpredictable variance in flavor/texture, but there are many processed foods that are high in fiber, such as fiber bars. Many favorite food items, such as refined wheat pasta, can potentially be swapped for higher-fiber pasta, like lentil pasta. If your child craves the familiar predictability of processed food items, try to find some that your child will eat while also helping to meet nutritional needs.

4. Make sure your child is stable on the toilet and explore good elimination positions. Try a "squatty potty" if your child prefers to squat while pooping.

5. Read stories about pooping to ease their anxieties and fears such as, *It Hurts When I Poop! A Story for Children Who Are Scared to use the Toilet* by Howard J. Bennett and *A Feel Better Book for Little Poopers* by Leah Bowen, Holly Brochmann and Shirley Ng-Benitez (illustrator).

Unfortunately, constipation might be an ongoing problem with your ASD child. But instead of considering medicine and intrusive measures to bring about consistent and comfortable bowel movements, it's more important to discover why your child has constipation. Once you know why your child is regularly constipated, you can find ways to naturally correct the problem.

Poor Interoceptive Awareness

Interoceptive awareness is the ability to physically sense when your bladder is full or when you need to have a bowel movement. Unfortunately, individuals with autism tend to have poor interoceptive awareness and therefore don't always know when they need to use the toilet until it's too late. This is especially true of younger children with autism. When an individual doesn't recognize the need to go, accidents will happen.

Parents of children with ASD may successfully toilet train their child, but the lack of interoceptive awareness may result in constant accidents and soiling. The best way to avoid these accidents during the toileting process is to train your child to habitually go to the bathroom every two to three hours. By scheduling toilet time, you have more of a chance to catch them when they truly need to go. As they get older and develop better interoceptive awareness, they will learn to identify when they need to use the toilet.

Fecal Smearing

It's not uncommon for an individual who is constipated or actively withholding bowel movements to display fecal smearing. Caregivers, teachers, and parents may assume this is a behavioral problem and that the child is purposely doing this because they are angry, upset, or expressing refusal to eliminate in the toilet. But fecal smearing is often more a result of constipation and withholding.

Reasons for Fecal Smearing

The hard fecal matter building up in the bowel due to constipation becomes uncomfortable, itchy, or even painful. When that happens, in order to feel some relief or to remove the feces, a child might use their fingers to dig out what they can. With feces now on their fingers and hands, the child will often smear it on the toilet, the walls, the floor, or clothing to remove it.

If your child is smearing feces, suspect constipation and treat the constipation. If you think your child is withholding, address that issue immediately. Above all, talk to your child about this very inappropriate and unhygienic behavior and teach your child the rules regarding fecal matter.

If constipation isn't the issue, your child may have problems using toilet paper and wiping appropriately. Sometimes as kids attempt to use toilet paper, poop gets on their fingers or hand. Watch your child as they use toilet paper and make sure they are doing it properly, then teach them to use more toilet paper and to fold the toilet paper before using it. Folding the toilet paper will prevent the paper from tearing and the children getting feces on their hands.

If smearing feces without intent gets a big, negative reaction from adults, then the child may do it again to gain attention or to get a big, negative reaction. If you suspect this is the cause of fecal smearing, always remain calm when it happens and relay the consequences of the fecal smearing. In these cases, make the child help to clean up the feces, and if the smearing continues, reward them for NOT smearing feces.

Addressing Fecal Smearing

Explain to your child that:
1. Poop needs to go in the toilet. This is the rule.
2. We use toilet paper to wipe poop off our bottoms.
3. Feces (poop) is very dirty and should not be smeared on anything!
4. If poop gets on our hands, we can use a wet wipe to clean off hands while sitting on the toilet (parents may need to

provide wet wipes if feces often gets on a child's hands and to prevent smearing). If the toilet can tolerate wet wipes, have the child drop the dirty wipe in the toilet after using.

5. We always wash our hands very well with soap and water after using the toilet and especially well if we get feces (poop) on our fingers and hands. When washing off feces, make sure the whole hand and under fingernails are clean of poop.

6. If feces gets on anything (walls, floor, toilet, etc.) it must be cleaned up right away. With adult supervision, have your child help with the cleaning, even if their help is minimal.

7. Anytime feces gets on something because of smearing, they must tell mom or dad and help to clean it up.

Aggression and Retaliation

Some children, especially older ones, will fight using the toilet and find ways to sabotage the process. Aggression toward others and destruction of property are common ways for them to express their anger and fear. Purposeful urinating and defecating in places other than the toilet may also occur.

These types of actions can really test the resolve of any parent. It is also hard to remain calm and encouraging under those circumstances, but that is exactly what you need to do. Instead of giving up the toilet training, it's important to think about what is triggering the anger and fear in your child. If necessary, take a step back to a task your child can comfortably do. Then, while using an appropriate means of communicating with your child, determine what is upsetting him/her.

Calmly explain that it's okay to be upset sometimes, but it's not okay to hurt others or damage property. Help them communicate their anger and fear and talk through a solution, with an emphasis on encouragement. A Social Story™, written about a specific anxiety, anger, or fear they may have will help them manage their emotions.

If they do any damage or intentionally eliminate, making a mess in their underwear or in places other than the toilet, remind them that they need to be responsible for helping to clean the mess. Cleaning up a mess they made, even partially participating in the cleanup, should be an expectation for your child, especially for older children.

Avoid punishing aggression, but remind them that no rewards will be given for bad behavior. On the other hand, tell them they will be rewarded for cooperative behavior and for trying their best.

TIPS AND STRATEGIES TO REMEMBER:

- Withholding is a serious, medical problem. If a child is withholding, find out why, adjust your toileting plan, and seek medical assistance if it continues.
- There are many reasons a person with ASD is withholding bowel movements or urine, as mentioned in this chapter. No matter the reason, withholding can cause long-lasting, physical problems and should be addressed immediately.
- Constipation is one of the most common bowel problems for people with ASD and is often a reason for withholding.
- There are several symptoms of and contributing factors to constipation listed in this chapter, which parents and school staff should be aware of.
- Constipation and the medical treatment of it can be traumatic for a child. Read through the natural constipation treatments in this chapter for easier ways to address it.

- If a child with ASD has poor interoceptive awareness, get them in the habit of using a toilet every two to three hours until they achieve better bladder and bowel awareness.
- Fecal smearing is often connected to severe constipation. It can also be a result of poor toilet paper use or as a means of negative attention-seeking.
- No matter the reason for fecal smearing, deal with it the same way by explaining the rules and consequences whenever fecal smearing occurs. Individuals who smear feces need to be made responsible for any fecal smearing.
- While trying to toilet train, whenever an adult is faced with aggression and sabotage by an individual, they should respond calmly, explain the rules, and make the child take responsibility for any damage they make. Remind the child that there are rewards for good behavior. A Social Story™ that addresses anger and aggression would be a good way to help curb aggressive outbursts.

Diapers to Underpants

Transitioning

Going from wearing diapers to wearing underwear is a major change for a child. Diapers look and feel different from underpants, and there is now the responsibility of learning to pull down or remove underpants when using the toilet or getting dressed and undressed. Some children transition easily to wearing underwear, while others, especially those with sensory sensitivities, may dislike the feel of underpants and will resist wearing them. If a child refuses to wear underpants, parents need to find out why. It could be the feel of the fabric, the color or design of the underwear, the tightness of the elastic waist, or something else. To the best of their ability, parents need to find out why their child refuses or resists wearing underpants and make changes to fit the needs of their child. Children will often take off underpants that get wet with urine or other liquid. Likewise, if a child soils their underwear, they will also want to remove it. Expect that anytime underwear feels uncomfortable, a child is likely to want it off.

Consider using training pants before making the immediate transition from diapers to underpants. Training pants are often used to help kids learn to use underpants while also catching any possible little accidents in their underwear. Training pants are thicker and may resemble the feel of diapers on a child, but like with underpants, a child will feel the wetness if they pee in them.

There have been cases of children who so dislike underwear that they choose not to wear it at all. This can be problematic at school or in public, especially as children enter puberty. It's important to help children transition to underpants and find the kind they like and will wear.

Steps to Successfully Wearing Underpants

1. When shopping for underwear, always allow a child to choose their own. Allow them to decide what kind they want, including the color and design.
2. Have your child decide which type of underpants they like: boxers, briefs, or boxer briefs for boys, and bikini or waist-high underpants for girls. They may need to try a variety of underpants before deciding which kind they like.
3. Show your child how to wear the underwear. Underwear worn backwards can feel uncomfortable. Teach them how to put it on and take it off.
4. If your child still needs to have and feel thicker underpants, consider using training pants before transitioning to standard underwear.
5. If your child can't tolerate the feel of the underpants, consider

washing it a few times to soften it up. If that doesn't work, look for underpants made with more tolerable fabric.

6. If you can't determine why your child doesn't like underwear, use their communication system to figure out the problem: too tight? Too scratchy? Too loose? Too light? Too confining? Whatever the reason, it's important you discover the problem to find the underpants your child will willingly wear.

7. Once you find the perfect underwear for your child, use only that kind until your child decides they want a change.

TIPS AND STRATEGIES TO REMEMBER:

- Diapers to underpants is a big change for kids with ASD. Consider transitioning to softer, bulkier training pants first.
- If your child hates underpants, find out why (using a communication board or device) and resolve the problem.
- Always allow your child to pick their own underpants.
- Teach your child the appropriate way to pull underpants off and on when they use the toilet. Boys who are learning to use the urinal need to learn how to pull the front of the underpants down without pulling down the backs of their pants and underpants.

Nighttime Toilet Training

Problems Associated with Night Training

Learning to wake up and go to the bathroom when needed is probably the last hurdle in toilet training. Night training isn't achieved until day training and the awareness of a full bladder or bowel occurs. For many kids with ASD, it may take a long time to achieve the goal of staying dry and accident-free during the night, even when they are successful using the toilet during the day.

Medication may contribute to nighttime accidents. Medication is often prescribed to people with autism, and certain medications can affect sleep patterns. Children with ASD often have difficulty sleeping and may require medication to sleep or relax. Such a medication may result in heavy or deep sleep and may inhibit a person's ability to wake up when they need to go to the bathroom.

Poor interoceptive awareness, also typical of youngsters with autism, dulls their ability to sense when their bladder is full and they need to move their bowels. This becomes especially problematic if your child is a deep sleeper and unaware of the need to wake up and go to the bathroom.

Taking Precautions

It may take years after your child has been successfully day-trained to use the toilet before your child is fully nighttime-trained as well. Until that maturity and awareness occurs, parents may choose to keep their child in diapers during the night and take actions to limit urine damage to the bed and mattress.

Even older children and adults with ASD who are completely toilet-trained may experience the occasional accident in bed. Some older individuals with autism find setting an alarm to wake up in the middle of the night to get up and use the toilet prevents bedwetting.

It may be necessary to keep a child in diapers or nighttime pull-ups at bedtime. Parents should also take measures to protect the bed, such as with plastic mattress covers. Nighttime training is often a long and slow process for all kids, whether they have autism or not. And even after they are successfully nighttime-trained, occasional accidents will likely occur. No matter the measures you take, continue to help your child remain dry at night to the best of their ability, and let them know that staying dry and diaper-free is the ultimate goal.

Contributing Factors for Nighttime Wetting

1. Drinking too much before bedtime
2. Not using the toilet just before going to bed

3. Not using the toilet first thing when waking up
4. Medication which causes heavy sleeping
5. Constipation
6. Poor interoceptive awareness (the inability to feel their full bladder)
7. Stress and anxiety

It's important that kids who are prone to wetting the bed stop drinking liquids one to two hours before bedtime. They should always use the toilet just before bed and immediately after waking up.

Remember to be patient but persistent when night-training your child. Anticipate and plan for accidents, as they will no doubt happen. As always, encourage your child and reward them for following the nighttime routine, even if bedwetting occurs.

TIPS AND STRATEGIES TO REMEMBER:

- Nighttime training takes longer than daytime training. Take precautions at night and expect bedtime accidents.
- Be aware of any contributing factors to nighttime wetting (see above) and manage them.
- Despite nighttime accidents, continue to be encouraging and let your child know that even if they have occasional accidents, they will be rewarded for following the bedtime routine and going potty before bedtime and as soon as they wake up.

Support Stories

Writing Support Stories

The stories included in this book are technically not Social Stories™, which follow a very specific formula, but are support stories written in a similar style as a Social Story™. These support stories are exceptionally helpful in preparing your child for the expectations of using the toilet. These support stories describe the situations in a way that a child will understand, while also explaining the rules and steps to be followed. Furthermore, these stories help to make the experience more personal by including your child's feelings and possible fears.

Support stories and generic stories that are similar to Social Stories™ have been proven to be very helpful for children with autism. These stories prepare someone with autism for an event or activity. The stories help them to understand what is happening and to accept the changes that will occur. The stories can give step-by-step instructions for the child to follow while considering the child's feelings and behaviors during the activity described in the support story.

Most of these support stories are written in the first person to make it more affirmative and personal. When using these stories with an individual child, include the child's actual name in the story. In this way, the story becomes the child's story and speaks for the individual child.

When writing a supportive teaching story, keep the language and vocabulary simple so that your child will easily understand it. Use line-drawn pictures or photos to illustrate your story. Illustrations are especially needed to help your child understand and remember the information, as well as to make the story more personal and interesting. If your child is already using and understanding a picture system, use those pictures to illustrate your stories. If your child needs photos to understand a situation, look online to find appropriate photos to use in your stories. Ask your child's school for picture resources, if necessary. You can also ask the school to help you make the stories for your child if that's something they can do for you.

Parents or teachers can also create stories together with the child. The adult can begin with asking the child questions about how they feel about using the toilet, while focusing on the specific concerns your child may have. We need to listen to children when they clearly communicate their fears, anxiety, and anger when it comes to using the toilet. Children might communicate verbally or behaviorally; regardless, we need to pay attention to what they are telling us. Children who have the language skills to tell us why they can't or won't use the toilet need to have their concerns considered. Remember to use what they tell you in the stories you both create.

The following generic support stories are samples you can use with your child or student. These stories can be rewritten with your child's name and picture and used to help your son or daughter with the toileting process. Most of these stories are long, but can be broken down into two or more stories as needed. For younger children and those who have a harder time understanding information, break the longer stories into two or three smaller ones, focusing on one topic with limited content per story.

Read the personalized stories aloud to your child while pointing to the pictures. Take your time and read the story more than once. As you make progress with the toilet, you can even create more specific support stories or Social Stories™ together with your child.

When creating your personalized story, use your child's words for urination and defecation. In the following stories, I use the words "pee" and "poop." If your child doesn't understand or use those words, change them to the ones your child uses.

TIPS AND STRATEGIES TO REMEMBER:

- When creating a support story, illustrate with pictures your child understands, and personalize the story for them.
- Keep the language simple and topic specific. Some children can handle more than one topic per story, but most will get confused and overwhelmed with too much information.
- Listen to your child and take their fears, sensitivities, and concerns into account when you create a support story or a Social Story™.
- Write each story with your child, if possible.
- Read the story with your child several times, as needed.
- Be prepared to write more support stories as new situations come up.

Sample Generic
Support Stories

People Use the Toilet

The toilet is an important part of the house because people use the toilet every day.

I can see my toilet in the bathroom. The bathroom is the room where the toilet belongs.

People use the toilet to pee and poop. Mom and Dad and my family use the toilet to pee and poop.

First, people take off their pants and underpants then sit on the toilet seat to pee and poop. The pee and poop go into the toilet bowl.

When people are finished peeing and pooping, they wipe their bottoms with toilet paper.

The toilet paper is used to clean and dry their bottoms. When someone is finished using the toilet paper, the dirty/wet toilet paper is dropped in the toilet.

After using the toilet, people press down the handle on the toilet to flush the pee, poop, and toilet paper down the toilet drain.

Using the toilet looks easy, and someday I will be able to use the toilet too.

The toilet may be scary and hard for me to use now, but soon I will learn to use the toilet just like everyone else.

When I learn to use the toilet, I will be brave and try my best. Mom and Dad will help me learn to use the toilet, and I will do a good job. I want to use the toilet, just like everyone else!

Many People Like to Use the Toilet

Many people like to sit on the toilet seat to do their business, but men and boys will usually stand and face the toilet when they pee because it is faster and easier.

Men and boys need to watch carefully to make sure their pee goes into the toilet and not on the floor. If I (a boy) stand to pee in the toilet, I will make sure my pee goes into the toilet. I think I will like standing and peeing in the toilet!

It's easy to use the toilet. Using the toilet is a quick and clean way to pee and poop. That's why lots of people like to use the toilet.

If a toilet is too big or uncomfortable for me, I can sit on a potty chair. A potty chair looks like a little toilet and is very easy to use. I can use a potty chair until I am big enough to use the toilet.

Soon I will use the toilet just like Mom, Dad, and other people. When I learn to use the toilet, I will be able to use the toilet whenever I need to. I will be able to go potty all by myself when I use a toilet. Using the toilet means I am a big girl/boy!

I Can Wear Diapers in the Bathroom

I'm not ready to pee or poop without diapers yet. I still need a diaper to feel ready to pee or poop. Peeing or pooping on the toilet without a diaper is just too hard!

I know when I need to pee or poop and will ask Mom or Dad for a diaper. Once I'm wearing a diaper, I feel comfortable and ready to pee or poop.

The bathroom is the place to pee and poop. Everyone is supposed to pee or poop in the bathroom because that's where pee and poop belong.

Even though I still need a diaper, I will do my business and pee and poop in the bathroom.

Once I'm done doing my business in my diaper, Mom or Dad can help me take it off, and I will dump my poop from the diaper into the toilet.

Poop belongs in the toilet, and I can do a good job putting it in there.

After I'm done dumping my poop in the toilet, I will flush the toilet and wash my hands.

I'm learning to do a good job in the bathroom, and soon I'll be ready to pee and poop in the toilet without a diaper!

The Toilet is Sometimes Scary

I don't like the toilet because it's sometimes scary. It makes a loud flushing noise, which is scary to hear.

When the toilet flushes, the water inside swirls around fast then goes down the hole at the bottom.

Anything that goes into the toilet gets sucked quickly down the large hole.

Things that get flushed into the toilet go away and never come back. I'm afraid I will get sucked into the toilet and not be able to get back! I'm afraid I could go down the toilet and be gone forever.

But my parents and adults tell me that can never happen. I'm too big to go down the toilet, even if I accidentally fall in the toilet. I know I will not get flushed down the toilet.

It's sometimes scary to sit on the toilet, but I know I won't go down the drain. I can do a good job peeing and pooping in the toilet, where my pee and poop can go down the drain. Yay!

A Toilet is Like a Big Drain

The toilet is like a big drain, only noisier. Water goes down the toilet just like water goes down the bathtub or sink drain.

Only pee, poop, and toilet paper should go in the toilet. Sometimes adults put other things in the toilet to clean it, but I should not put anything in the toilet that doesn't belong there.

We want to flush the smelly pee, poop, and dirty toilet paper down the toilet. That's where pee, poop and dirty toilet paper belong.

Because the hole in the toilet is big, we need to be careful not to drop things in the toilet that don't belong there. We don't want to clog the toilet with too much toilet paper or other things that don't belong there.

I know that the toilet is just a big, noisy drain with water in it. I know that a toilet is important for getting rid of pee, poop, and dirty toilet paper. I know that I'm too big to go down the toilet, and that's a good thing!

The toilet looks and sounds scary, but I know it's just a big drain for pee, poop, and toilet paper. It's not scary anymore.

Soon I will learn to use the toilet like Mommy and Daddy and other people. I used to be afraid of the toilet, but now I'm not. I know I will be able to do a good job using the toilet.

I Can Sit on the Potty Chair

I have been wearing diapers for a long time, ever since I was a baby. But now I'm a big boy (or girl) and it's time for me to use the potty chair instead of wearing diapers.

Sitting on the potty chair and peeing and pooping is a big change for me. But it doesn't hurt to sit on the potty chair, and I will do a good job trying to use the potty chair instead of diapers.

I will need to sit on the potty chair without a diaper. It will feel strange to sit on the potty chair because it has a large hole for the pee and poop to go in. It will feel strange at first, but soon I will get used to it.

I only need to sit on the potty chair for a short time. I don't need to sit until I pee or poop; that will happen later when I'm comfortable sitting on the potty chair.

Soon I will feel comfortable sitting on the potty chair and soon I will be able to pee and poop in the potty chair.

I will do a good job sitting on the potty chair, and I will feel proud when I'm able to do it all by myself.

I Like My Potty Chair, But Now
I Need to Use the Big Toilet

I like my potty chair, and I can use the potty chair all by myself.

I like my potty chair because it's small and comfortable. It's easy to sit on my potty chair.

But now I'm getting bigger, and the potty chair is too small for me to use.

Mom and Dad say I need to start using the big toilet.

I'm a little afraid to use the big toilet because it's hard to sit on and the opening is large.

The big toilet is full of water and noisy when it flushes.

I know I need to use the big toilet because everywhere I go, there will only be big toilets for me to use to go potty.

When I need to go potty at school, I will have to use a big toilet.

Until I get comfortable using a big toilet, I can have a nice toilet seat insert, which will be easy to sit on and make it feel like a small toilet.

It will be hard to change from using a potty chair to using a big toilet, but I know I can do it.

Soon I will be able to use a big toilet like Mom and Dad and everyone I know. I'm a big boy (girl) and I can use a big toilet!

Mommy (Daddy) Will Help Me
Learn to Use the Potty

I don't need to use the toilet (potty chair) by myself. Mommy and Daddy will help me.

Mommy will tell me when it's time to sit on the potty chair and try to pee or poop. Mommy will help me and tell me I'm doing a good job.

Sometimes I may feel afraid and upset to use the toilet. It's okay to feel upset and afraid at first. If I'm afraid of the toilet (potty chair), I will tell Mommy. Mommy will listen to me when I'm scared and upset. Mommy and daddy will help me feel better.

Using the potty chair may be hard at first, but Mommy and Daddy will help me, and they will give me special treats and surprises when I do a good job trying to use the potty chair.

I will do a good job trying to use the potty chair. I will do a good job and then I will earn special treats.

Anxiety Can Make Me Feel
Scared and Upset

Sometimes when I think about using the potty (toilet), I get scared and upset and I don't feel right.

My heart may beat very fast, and I will feel sweaty and panicked. I might even feel dizzy and sick.

This feeling is called anxiety, and having anxiety might make me feel like I want to run away or hide. I may have scary thoughts that I can't stop.

When I'm anxious and panicked, I feel out of control and can't seem to calm down.

Feeling anxious (having anxiety) might make me so scared that when people try to help me, I sometimes hurt them or try to keep them away from me.

I know that many things can make me feel anxious and upset, including using the toilet.

I don't like feeling anxious and out of control, but I usually don't know how to stop it.

Adults can help me when I feel anxious and upset. Adults can help me find ways to calm down and feel better.

Whenever I feel anxious and upset, I need to tell Mom and Dad and all my teachers. Adults will help me learn how to calm down.

I don't like feeling anxious and upset. I want to feel calm. I know I need to tell adults when I'm anxious and upset, and they will know what to do to make me feel better. Anxious feelings won't last forever, and soon I can be calm again.

I will learn ways to calm down, and I will do a good job calming down whenever I feel anxious. I like to feel calm!

Thinking About Using the Toilet Makes Me Anxious and Upset

A lot of things, like using the toilet, make me feel anxious and upset. When there's a change or something new and unexpected, I might get anxious and upset.

Using the toilet is a big change for me. And when I need to learn a new or scary task, like using the potty, I know I will get anxious.

Thinking about using the toilet makes me anxious and upset, and I don't like feeling scared and anxious!

I need to tell my mom, dad, and my teachers when I'm anxious and upset. My mom, dad, and teachers will help me find strategies to calm down.

I can ask for sensory toys to help me calm down.

I can look at my list of calming strategies to find one(s) to calm me down.

I can ask for more strategies to help me get calm.

If I feel too anxious, I can ask for a break and leave the bathroom.

I can leave the bathroom to calm down and when I'm ready, I can try to use the toilet again. I know adults can help me calm down.

Soon, learning to use the toilet won't be scary and I won't feel anxious. I know adults will help me not feel scared. I know I can do a good job calming down and using the toilet.

I Want to Feel Calm When
I Use the Potty (Toilet)

Learning to use the potty can make me feel anxious and upset, but my parents and teachers can help me get calm again. I need to trust my parents and teachers to find ways to make me feel calm and ready to do something new.

My parents and teachers will help me find things I can do to make my anxiety go away and help me be calm again, so that I can calmly learn to use the potty/toilet.

Adults can help me find strategies to calm me down when I get upset. I can use the strategies that work best for me.

If I know I'm feeling anxious and upset, I need to tell my teachers and parents so they can help me. I will use my list of calming strategies to help me feel better.

I can try ways to get calm and find the ones that work best for me. Getting calm can sometimes be hard, but if I find the ways that work for me and practice getting calm, I can do a good job and feel better.

When my anxious thoughts and feelings are gone, I can do a good job learning to use the potty/toilet.

Learning to use the toilet is important. I know I can get calm and do a good job using the toilet. I will trust adults to help me find ways to get calm.

I Don't Want to Feel Uncomfortable
in the Bathroom

There are many reasons to be uncomfortable in the bathroom and when I'm using the toilet.

Sometimes people don't like the smells in the bathroom. Sometimes the lights bother them or they don't like the sounds of the exhaust fans or the toilet flushing. Lots of things bother me in the bathroom.

Sometimes I might not like the feeling of sitting on the toilet with a bare bottom. Sometimes it feels cold or too hard. Maybe it's because I feel too exposed and don't like the feeling of water splashing on my bottom.

If I don't like something in the bathroom or the toilet, I need to tell or show my parents or teachers. Parents and adults who help me won't know if something is bothering me unless I tell them. I need to tell adults when something in the bathroom bothers me.

Something might really bother me, like lights or sounds or smells, which don't bother anyone else. Sometimes parents, teachers, and other kids don't even notice the things that really bother me.

If I can't handle the bright lights, or toilet and fan noises, I need to tell Mommy and Daddy. If anything in the bathroom bothers me, I need to tell someone. My parents or other adults will know how to fix it for me.

I won't scream or fight when something is bothering me. Instead, I will tell an adult what is bothering me. I can ask for a break or for a sensory toy to help me.

Whatever the problem is, I know I can tell adults and they will help me.

I know I can use the toilet and do a good job when I feel comfortable in the bathroom and on the toilet.

I Get Distracted in the Bathroom

I like being in the bathroom because there are lots of things to see, hear, smell and touch.

It's hard for me to pay attention to what I'm supposed to do in the bathroom because I want to pay attention to other things. I want to do things I want to do.

Sometimes I want to look at the flickering lights or listen to the exhaust fan. Sometimes lots of interesting smells distract me. And sometimes I want to touch things I shouldn't touch or wash my hands over and over.

Sometimes I want to do things over and over again and I just can't stop. It might be part of my own routine or something I just like to do.

My parents and other adults might get upset because I don't want to do what they ask me to do. Sometimes they get upset because I ignore them.

I know if I do a good job and pay attention to what adults want me to do, I can get a reward. I like getting rewards, and sometimes the rewards will be doing the things I want to do in the bathroom.

I know I need to pay attention to what adults want me to do in the bathroom. I know I need to do a good job using the toilet and following the bathroom rules.

I will let adults know when I'm distracted, and I will try my best to stay focused and earn rewards.

I want to do a good job in the bathroom and earn rewards. I will follow the rules and do a good job!

I Will Try My Best to Use the Toilet

Sometimes I get very upset when I must sit on the toilet. Sitting on the toilet sometimes makes me feel sad, angry, and upset.

I get so upset that I can't go in the toilet. I get so upset that I get angry and want to hurt someone and break things.

It's okay to get upset, but it's not okay to hurt anyone or break things.

When I get upset about using the toilet, I need to tell Mom, Dad, or another adult. When I let them know that I'm upset, they will help me fix what is bothering me and feel better.

Sometimes I have a hard time using the toilet because I was doing something else, and I didn't want to stop what I was doing. Changing from one activity to another is hard for me.

Sometimes I don't want to sit on the toilet because I don't know how long I must sit.

Sometimes I don't want to sit on the toilet because I don't want or need to go potty.

Sometimes I don't know why I'm upset sitting on the toilet. But no matter why I'm upset, I must show or tell an adult, so they can fix it.

I know that sitting on the toilet is about learning to pee or poop in the toilet.

I know I need to practice trying to go in the toilet.

I need to let adults know when I'm sad, mad, or upset about using the toilet. Mom, Dad, and other adults can help me feel calm so I can do a good job when I sit on the toilet.

Adults will prepare me for using the toilet and will tell me how long I need to sit. Adults will help me relax so I can do a good job.

When I do a good job sitting on the toilet, I can get a reward. I will try my best to sit on the toilet. I know I can do a good job when I try my best.

Rewards Are the Best!

Everyone likes getting rewards. I like getting rewards, too! Rewards are the best!

Every time I pee or poop in the potty chair (toilet) I will get a reward. Rewards are fun, exciting, and sometimes surprising! I like getting rewards!

Sometimes I might get a yummy treat to eat. Sometimes I might get a toy or something fun to do. I know if I do a good job using the potty chair, I will get a reward.

Sometimes I like getting the same reward. And sometimes I like getting different rewards. Sometimes I will get surprise rewards. I can choose which rewards I want to get. I love getting rewards!

All I have to do is try my best to pee and poop in the potty chair (toilet) and then I can get a reward. Mommy (Daddy) and my teachers will help me earn rewards.

Sometimes it's hard and scary to pee and poop in the potty chair, but I will try my best. I know if I do a good job, I will get a reward, and rewards are the best!

I'm Not Afraid to Poop in the Toilet

I'm a big boy (girl) and I need to go poop in the toilet. Mommy and Daddy, my siblings, and everyone I know go poop in the toilet. They aren't afraid to poop in the toilet. I will learn to poop in the toilet too, and I won't be afraid.

Poop belongs in the toilet. When I need to go poop, I won't make a mess in my pants. I will go to the bathroom and let my poop go into the toilet (potty chair) where it belongs.

Pooping in the toilet may feel different and strange, but I know I'm okay and it doesn't hurt to poop in the toilet. I won't be afraid to poop in the toilet.

When I feel like poop needs to come out, I will sit on the toilet (potty chair) and wait for the poop to come out.

Sometimes when I sit on the toilet, my poop doesn't come out right away. Sometimes I need to relax and think about other things or look at a book before my poop is ready to come out. It's okay to wait until I feel comfortable for my poop to come out.

Even though it may feel a little scary and strange to let poop fall into the toilet, I will do a good job and not try to stop the poop from coming out. I won't be afraid to poop in the toilet.

Pooping in the toilet feels strange and different, but I know it will get better. Soon I will feel good pooping in the toilet. Pooping in the toilet is easy! Soon I will feel proud about doing a good job pooping in the toilet.

I'm a big boy (girl)! I can poop in the toilet just like everyone else!

Pooping in the Toilet Feels Funny

Pooping in a toilet feels different from pooping in a diaper.

When I sit on a toilet or potty chair and poop comes out, it might feel like something is coming out of my body. It might feel wrong and scary!

But it isn't wrong, and it isn't scary. That's just how poop feels when it comes out.

It might feel strange at first, but soon I will get used to it, and it won't feel strange and scary anymore. I need to let the poop fall out of me into the toilet.

It's important that I let the poop out every day. If I don't let the poop out, my tummy will hurt, and it will hurt to poop if I wait too long.

My body needs to poop every day! I will do a good job letting my poop out in the toilet every day.

Going Potty is Something We All Have to Do

Going potty isn't a choice. We all need to go potty every day.

Going potty is something our body needs to do every day, like eating, drinking, and sleeping. Our bodies need to go potty every day.

If I don't go potty, I will get sick, and my body will hurt and feel bad.

I might be too busy to go potty maybe I just don't want to go. But waiting too long to go potty will make me feel sick and can cause an accident.

My body needs to go potty four or five times a day, and sometimes more. Going potty will make my body feel good and keep me healthy.

Sometimes if I forget to go potty, I might pee or poop in my pants. That makes a big mess!

My body decides when I need to go pee or poop. My body will tell me when I need to go, and I need to pay attention to the signals my body gives me that says I need to go potty.

Going potty is very important and I will remember to pay attention to my body and go potty four or five times every day.

I Don't Want Hard Poops!

Hard poops are uncomfortable and sometimes hurt. I don't like sitting on the toilet when I have hard poops.

Sometimes I need to poop, but I can't because my poop is too hard to come out.

Sometimes I'm afraid to go potty because I know my poop will hurt when I try to go.

I want to have softer poops. Softer poops come out easily and don't hurt.

I know I need to drink lots of water and eat some fruits and vegetables if I want soft poops. Sometimes I can drink juice to help me have soft poops.

Soft poops are better for my body. They come out easily when I need to go, and they won't hurt.

I don't like lots of fruits and vegetables, but I will find some that I like and eat them every day. Eating fruits and vegetables will give me good, soft poops.

I sometimes don't like to drink water, but I know drinking lots of water and juice will help me pee more and have softer poops.

Drinking lots of water and eating fruits and vegetables are good for my body.

I will do a good job drinking water and eating fruits and vegetables every day, and I will have soft, easy poops.

Sometimes I Can't Go Poop

Sometimes I can't go poop because it's too hard and it hurts to poop.

Sometimes I don't want to poop because I'm worried or afraid.

If I'm worried and afraid to poop, I need to tell Mommy or Daddy.

Poop always needs to come out. I should not try to hold my poop in.

Holding my poop in will make it hurt even more when the poop finally comes out.

Holding my poop in will make me sick and will hurt me.

If I can't poop because it's too hard or it hurts to poop, I must always tell Mommy or Daddy.

I need to remember that poop always needs to come out.

If I don't poop and Mommy and Daddy can't help me poop, I may need to go to a doctor to help me poop. Because poop always needs to come out.

I will always try to let my poop out, but if it's too hard for me to poop, I will tell Mommy and Daddy and anyone who takes care of me that I need help.

Using Toilet Paper

We use toilet paper to keep our bottoms clean and dry after we use the toilet or potty chair.

We need to use toilet paper every time we sit on the toilet or potty chair and pee or poop. We can use a few squares of toilet paper when we pee, and maybe more squares, about four or five when we poop.

Wiping my front once with a few squares of toilet paper should be enough to dry myself after I pee. I always drop the wet toilet paper in the toilet or potty chair when I'm finished wiping.

I may need to wipe myself more than once when I poop. I may need to wipe myself two or more times with more toilet paper each time to be sure my bottom is clean after I poop.

Each time I use toilet paper to clean my bottom, I drop it in the toilet. Used toilet paper always belongs in the toilet. I just need to be sure not to put too much toilet paper in the toilet before flushing. Too much toilet paper can cause the toilet to clog up.

After I wipe myself with toilet paper, I will flush the toilet and wash my hands with soap and water.

I Don't Wear Diapers

When I was a baby and little, I wore diapers.

But now that I'm big and use the toilet, I don't need to wear diapers.

Diapers are only for kids who don't use the toilet yet to pee and poop.

When I learn to use the toilet all the time like big kids, I won't need to wear diapers.

It may be scary and upsetting to not wear diapers anymore. I only remember wearing diapers, so not wearing diapers will be a hard change for me.

But Mommy and Daddy will help me feel comfortable not wearing diapers.

Instead of diapers, I can wear underpants, which I can pick out myself. My underpants can be colorful and pretty, and I can look cool in my new underpants.

Mommy and Daddy and big kids don't wear diapers. They wear underpants. I won't need to wear diapers either. I can be a big kid wearing underwear.

Once I learn to use the toilet, I won't wear diapers, and no one will need to change my diapers.

It will feel strange and different to not wear diapers at first, but soon I will get used to wearing underpants, and I won't miss having diapers on.

I can go to the bathroom by myself without diapers. I can be private and independent in the bathroom when I don't wear diapers.

Not wearing diapers means I'm a big kid and I can use the toilet by myself!

I Know When I Need to Use the Toilet

Our bodies will let us know when we need to pee or poop. Our bodies will tell us when we need to use the toilet.

When I need to use the toilet, my bladder, the thing in my body that holds my pee, will feel full. I will feel uncomfortable, and a message will go to my brain that I need to go to the bathroom to pee.

Sometimes we can ignore the full feeling that means we need to pee. But we can't ignore it for too long! Soon we will need to quickly go to the bathroom to pee in the toilet.

I shouldn't ignore the feeling to pee, because if I wait too long to use the toilet, I will pee anyway. And I might pee in my pants! That will be a wet mess, and I will feel embarrassed!

I need to pay attention to my body, and I need to know when I should use the toilet. I should go to the bathroom before I'm too full of pee and I might have an accident.

My body will tell me when I need to pee.

- My bladder will feel full.
- I will feel uncomfortable.
- I might want to grab myself (which I shouldn't do around others).
- I might hop around because I need to pee.

When my body tells me to pee, I will pay attention and immediately go to the bathroom to pee in the toilet.

My body will also tell me when I need to poop.

134

- My bottom will feel full and heavy.
- I will feel uncomfortable.
- It will feel like poop is starting to come out.
- I might need to squeeze my bottom to hold it in.

When my body tells me that I need to poop, I will pay attention and immediately go to the bathroom and poop in the toilet.

If I don't pay attention to my body, I might poop in my pants and make a big mess. It will be stinky, messy, and embarrassing!

My body will tell me when I need to pee or poop. I will pay attention to my body, and I will know when I need to use the toilet.

I will do a good job and go to the bathroom before I get too full and have an accident!

Poop is Very Dirty!

Poop is very dirty, and I must try not to get it on my hands.

Whenever I try to wipe poop, I will use toilet paper. Toilet paper can help keep my hands clean when I'm wiping poop.

I won't try to touch poop with my fingers or hands because I know it is very dirty and gross!

I won't wipe poop on myself or the floor or the walls or the toilet or anything but toilet paper. Poop belongs in the toilet; I will wipe away any poop on myself with toilet paper.

If I accidentally get poop on my hands, I will first wipe my hands with toilet paper or wet wipe, then drop the dirty toilet paper (or wet wipe) in the toilet.

After I wipe my hands with toilet paper, I will wash my hands with soap and water. I will wash my hands and fingernails and make sure all the poop is off and that my hands and fingers are very clean.

I know that poop is very dirty and shouldn't go on anything but toilet paper. I will remember to do a good job using toilet paper when I wipe my poop.

I Use the Bathroom at School

I use the bathroom at school, and I can do a good job using the school bathroom all by myself.

If I need to use the toilet, I will go into a bathroom stall and close the door behind me for privacy.

The toilet at school will look different from my toilet at home, but that's okay. The toilet at school is still a toilet, and I can use it just like my toilet at home.

I will pull down my pants and underwear and sit on the toilet.

After I pee or poop, I will wipe my bottom with toilet paper. I don't need more than a few squares of toilet paper.

I will wipe from front to back and drop the dirty toilet paper into the toilet.

Sometimes, if my bottom is still dirty, I will wipe it again, until I notice that the toilet paper is clean. That shows me that I did a good job wiping my bottom.

I drop all the toilet paper I used in the toilet and flush the toilet.

I pull up my underwear and pants before I open the door and leave the stall.

After I leave the bathroom stall, I go to the bathroom sink and wash my hands with soap and water. It's important to have clean hands after using the toilet.

I dry my hands on a paper towel or use a hand air dryer until my hands are dry.

Now I'm ready to leave the bathroom. Good job!

Sometimes I Might Pee or Poop While I Sleep

If I need to go potty and I'm asleep, I might not know to wake up and go potty.

Sometimes at night or during a nap, I might pee or poop while I'm asleep.

If this happens, there will a mess in my bed and on my clothes.

This will make my bed feel wet and cold when I wake up.

I might have poop in my pajamas when I wake up.

My bed, my pajamas, and I will be a mess and will need to be cleaned up.

No one likes to pee and poop in bed, especially if it makes a mess.

I will remember to go potty right before I go to bed and as soon as I wake up in the morning. That will help me stay dry and clean at night.

I will remember not to drink too much water or other drinks just before bed. Drinking too much before bed will make me need to pee when I sleep.

If I wake up in the night, I will get up and go to the bathroom and go potty.

If I can't feel when I need to go potty at night and I don't wake up to go potty, I may need to wear a special diaper or pull-up at night.

I may need to wear a special diaper and pull-up only until I am able to wake up and go potty when I feel I need to.

I will do my best to go potty just before bed and as soon as I wake up in the morning. If I wake up at night and need to go potty, I will go right away to the bathroom.

It may take a long time to learn to wake up and go potty when I need to. Until I learn to go potty at night, I will do my best not to make a mess in my bed.

People Need Privacy in the Bathroom

Using a toilet is private. When people use the toilet, they will usually close the bathroom door to have privacy.

When I first learn to use the toilet, I will need help from Mom, Dad, and other adults. It may take me a long time to learn to use the toilet, but when I'm able to use the toilet without help, I will use the toilet privately by myself.

Mom and Dad, other adults, and big kids are private in the bathroom. I can learn to be private in the bathroom too.

When I can use the toilet all by myself, I will need privacy. I will go into the bathroom and shut the door.

When I can go potty by myself, I won't need anyone to help me, and no one needs to watch me use the toilet. Using the toilet should be private.

If I have a problem using the toilet and need help, I can always call out to Mom or another trusted adult to help me.

I will pull down my pants and sit on the toilet (or stand in front of the toilet). I will pee or poop and wipe myself with toilet paper when I'm done.

I will pull up my underpants and pants and flush the toilet. I can do all of this by myself.

Before leaving the bathroom, I will wash my hands with soap and water and dry them with a towel.

I can use the bathroom all by myself and I can have privacy in the bathroom. It's important to be private in the bathroom.

Using Different Bathrooms and Toilets

There are bathrooms and toilets almost everywhere. Some toilets look like the toilets I use, and some toilets and bathrooms will be different.

Toilets may look and smell and feel different, but they are all toilets which I can use to go pee or poop.

I might not like how a bathroom or toilet looks, feels, or smells, but if I need to go potty and it's the only bathroom to use, I will do my best to use it.

Sometimes I need to go potty immediately and can't wait to be home to use my own toilet or potty. Sometimes I need to use a different toilet.

It may be hard and uncomfortable to use a toilet I don't like, but I need to do my best. It's not okay to wet or make a mess in my pants because I don't want to use a different toilet.

Making a mess in my pants is a much bigger problem than using a different toilet. I don't want to make a mess in my pants!

If I don't like how a toilet looks or smells, I can wipe the seat or put toilet paper on the seat before I use it. I can hold my nose while using the toilet and pee and poop as quickly as possible!

Using a different bathroom and toilet might be hard and upsetting, but I will do my best to pee and poop in a toilet that I'm not used to.

It's important that I don't make a mess in my pants or try to stop my pee and poop for too long. It may be hard to use a toilet I don't like, but I know I can do it!

I will not make a mess in my pants, but instead I will do a good job using a different toilet.

Using a Urinal

Men and boys will sometimes use a urinal to pee. Sometimes when I pee, I might use a urinal.

I might see urinals in many different bathrooms. The bathrooms may look different, but most urinals look the same.

Urinals are easy to use. When I need to pee, I stand in front of the urinal, close enough to pee into it. I always stand to use a urinal. Urinals are not for sitting. And urinals are only for peeing.

I pull my pants and underwear down just enough to let me pee. I never drop my pants and underwear to the floor.

I can unzip my pants and open the fly of my underwear and pee into the urinal without taking my clothes off. I need to keep my backside covered.

I'm careful to only pee into the urinal and not on the floor. I will stand facing the urinal until I'm completely done peeing.

When I'm finished peeing, I will flush the urinal, pull up my underwear and pants, and go to the sink to wash my hands.

There Are Rules for Using a Urinal

Urinals are easy to use.

Many boys and men use urinals every day.

But urinals are not private, so there are rules for using them.

It's important to give someone using a urinal privacy.

When I go into a bathroom with many urinals, I need to use a urinal that isn't right next to a stranger using another urinal.

I need to give myself and any stranger using a urinal privacy.

When I use a urinal, I must remember not to drop my pants and underpants to the floor.

I need to give myself privacy by not showing my bare bottom to other people in the bathroom. This is very important!

I will only pull my pants and underpants down a little in the front to allow myself to pee.

While I'm in the bathroom, I must remember not to stare at men or boys using a urinal. I must give them privacy.

When I am using a urinal, I need to keep my eyes on my urinal and pay attention to what I'm doing. I won't look around or watch others using a urinal.

I will remember to only urinate in the urinal and not on the floor or wall. Peeing outside of the urinal is unsanitary, and other people in the bathroom will be disgusted if it happens.

Sometimes when a bathroom is crowded, I need to stand next to a stranger using a urinal. If that happens, I will remember to only look at my urinal and not look at the stranger peeing. I will be private and give the stranger privacy, too.

When I'm finished using my urinal, I will pull up my underwear and pants before I go to a sink to wash my hands with soap and water.

I will remember to be private and follow the urinal rules whenever I use a urinal in a bathroom with more than one urinal.

Sometimes I Might Have
an Accident in My Pants

I can use the toilet all by myself. But sometimes accidents happen.

I may be too busy to use the toilet and don't remember to go to the bathroom until it's too late.

I may need to use a toilet, but I can't find one to use.

I may be sick with diarrhea and not be able to control my pooping.

Maybe it hurts every time I pee, so I try not to.

I may really need to go to the bathroom, but I'm too far from a toilet.

Maybe I'm afraid to use a strange bathroom but can't hold my pee or poop until I find a familiar bathroom.

There are lots of reasons I could have an accident in my pants. And I'm not the only one who may sometimes have an accidental mess in my underpants. Almost everyone has had an occasional pee or poop accident in their pants, even adults.

If I sometimes wait too long to use the toilet, I will make sure I use the toilet as soon as I get the feeling I need to go. Waiting too long to use the toilet is risky and may cause an accident.

Sometimes it's important to plan ahead to avoid toileting accidents. If I know I won't be near a toilet for a long time, I will be sure to use a toilet before I'm far from one.

Even if I don't really need to pee, it's a good idea to use the bathroom before I go on a long car or bus ride, or if I know I won't be near any toilets for a while.

Sometimes strange bathrooms can be scary, and I might feel anxious. If I know I need to use a strange bathroom, I will take a friend or trusted adult with me, so I won't be alone in a strange bathroom.

If I have diarrhea and can't stop pooping, I will tell a parent or a trusted adult who can help me with that. Having diarrhea means I'm probably sick, and I really need to tell an adult when I'm sick.

If it hurts to pee, that means I might have an infection, and I must tell my parents and any adult caring for me.

If I feel like I need to pee all the time, that may also be a sign of an infection, and I will tell my parents and anyone taking care of me.

Toileting accidents sometimes happen. I will remember to not wait too long to use the toilet, and I will plan ahead if I know I won't have a toilet near me. Sometimes having extra underpants with me will help me be prepared in case I have an accident.

Any time I'm sick with diarrhea or an infection, I must tell my parents.

If I have a toileting accident in my pants, I won't get upset. I will tell a trusted adult and take care of it. Most toileting accidents can be prevented, and I will do my best to not have an accident in my pants.

Personalized Support Stories can be an excellent way to address specific issues regarding a child's toileting. But also consider reading a variety of kids' books about using the potty. There are many colorfully illustrated standard potty books for kids, which your son or daughter may find interesting and enjoyable. Consider going to the library or online to find the books your child may like. And allow your child to choose the books they enjoy reading.

Conclusion

When it comes to toilet training, just like learning any new skill, all children are different. Some will take to using the toilet easily, but others will have issues and take much longer. This manual serves to give various strategies and plans to address the possible difficulties children and parents may face. Hopefully this manual will provide both parents and teaching staff the answers to some questions and concerns regarding toileting, as well as the necessary strategies to tackle that task.

Above all, I urge parents and teachers to remain calm, encouraging, and persistent—and allow the toilet training of children (or even adults!) to occur at the individuals' pace. Don't give yourself a very rigid timeline to accomplish this goal—remember your long-term goal of your child one day being independent while using the toilet. How long it takes to arrive there is unimportant as long as progress continues. Small and slow steps forward are still steps forward!

Soon your child will be using the toilet on their own with confidence and independence. Remember, toilet training is a long, often hard, skill to acquire. But when your child masters the task of using the toilet independently, that's a huge accomplishment to be celebrated, with a lifetime of freedom and possibilities.

References, Resources & Additional Reading

Arnwine, Bonnie, and Olivia McCoy. *Starting Sensory Integration Therapy: Fun Activities That Won't Destroy Your Home*. Las Vegas: Sensory Resources, 2006.

Bennett, Howard. *Waking Up Dry: A Guide to Help Children Overcome Bedwetting*. American Psychological Association, 2005.

Beardon, Luke. *Avoiding Anxiety in Autistic Children: A Guide for Autistic Wellbeing (Overcoming Common Problems)*, London: Sheldon Press Hachette, 2021.

Chalfant, Anne M. *Managing Anxiety in People with Autism: A Treatment Guide for Parents, Teachers and Mental Health Professionals*. Woodbine House, Inc., 2011.

Delmolino, Lara. *Solve Common Teaching Challenges in Children with Autism: 8 Essential Strategies for Professionals & Parents*. Woodbine House, Inc., 2015.

Dubin, Nick. *Asperger Syndrome and Anxiety: A Guide to Successful Stress Management*, Kingsley Publishers, 2009.

Ferguson, Sophia J. *Stool Withholding-What To Do When Your Child Won't Poop!* Create Space Independent Publishing Platform, 2015.

Fleming, Eve and MacAlister, Lorraine. *Toilet Training and the Autism Spectrum: A Guide for Professionals*. United Kingdom: Jessica Kingsley Publishers, 2015.

Gray, Carol. *The Original Social Story™ Book*. Arlington, TX: Future Horizons, Inc., 1993.

Gray, Carol. *The New Social Story™ Book*. Arlington, TX: Future Horizons, Inc., 1994.

Hayden, Wendy. *What Your Doctor Didn't Tell You About Childhood Constipation*. Independently published, 2019.

Mouton-Odum, Suzanne. *Helping Your Child with Sensory Regulation: Skills to Manage the Emotional and Behavioral Components to Your Child's Sensory Processing Challenges*. Oakland, CA: New Harbinger Publications, 2021.

Wheeler, Maria. *Toilet Training for Individuals with Autism and Related Disorders*, Arlington, TX: A Comprehensive Guide for Parents and Teachers. Future Horizons, Inc., 1998.

Internet Resources

Aponte, Courtney and Mruzek, Daniel. *Seven Toilet Training Tips That Help Nonverbal Kids with Autism*. University of Rochester Medical Center, 2016. www.autismspeaks.org/blog.

Autism (ASD) and Sensory Processing Issues—Signs and How to Help. Griffin Occupational Therapy, 2019. https://www.griffinot.com/asd-and-sensory-processing-disorder/

Bennie, Maureen. *Constipation, Withholding, and Overflow—A Deeper Dive into Bowel Problems for Individuals with ASD*, 2020. https://autismawarenesscentre.com/constipation-witholding-and-overflow-a-deeper-dive-into-bowel-problems-for-individuals-with-asd/

https://autismawarenesscentre.com/the-difficulties-with-toilet-training-a-person-with-autism/

Bennie, Maureen. *The Difficulties with Toilet Training a Person with Autism*, 2019. https://autismawarenesscentre.com/the-difficulties-with-toilet-training-a-person-with-autism/

Ring, Rob. *Anxiety and Autism: How Common Are Anxiety Disorders*, Autism Speaks, Inc., 2019.
https://www.autismspeaks.org/expert-opinion/how-common-are-anxiety-disorders-people-autism

Williams, Shana. *Toilet Training the Child with Autism: Seven Tips for Parents*. Chatsworth, CA: California Psychcare, 2019.
https://360behavioralhealth.com/toilet-training-child-autism-7-tips/

Wood, Jeffery. *Managing Anxiety in Children with Autism*, Autism Speaks, Inc., 2014.
https://www.autismspeaks.org/expert-opinion/managing-anxiety-children-autism

Suggested Visual Supports

Boardmaker series of PCS symbols: Mayer-Johnson, Inc., www.mayer-johnson.com

Free Potty Training Visual Schedules (2018): www.andnextcomesl.com

Free Toileting Sequences for Autism: autismlittlelearners.com

Google Images: Toilet Instructions-Stock Photos and Shop Visual Supports for Teaching Toileting

Picture This ... Functional Living CD photos: Silver Lining Multimedia, Inc., www.silverliningmm.com

Toilet Training Autistic Children: In Pictures: raisingchildren.net.au

Toilet Training Visual Schedule: Pinterest, www.pinterest.com

Visual Aids for Learning-Toilet Training (Boy) NHS GGC: Downloadable sequence cards, www.nhsggc.org.uk

Visual Timetable Using the Toilet (Boys)—Twinkl: www.twinkl.com

Suggested Books for Children

It Hurts When I Poop! A Story for Children Who Are Scared to Use the Toilet by Howard J. Bennett (2007), American Psychological Association, publisher

A Feel Better Book for Little Poopers by Leeah Bonen and Holly Brochman. Illustrated by Shirley Ng-Benitez, (2020)

Everyone Poops by Taro Gomi. Chronicle Books, (2020)

Come Out Mr. Poo: Potty Training for Kids by Janelle McGuiness (2017)

Everyone Feels Anxious Sometimes by Dr. Daniela Owen (May 2021), Puppy Dogs & Ice cream, Inc. Other books by Daniela Owen include: *Everyone Feels Sad Sometimes* and *I Am Fine.*

I Can't, I Won't, No Way! A Book for Children Who Refuse to Poo by Tracey Vessillo (2011) Create Space Independent Publishing Platform.

About the Author

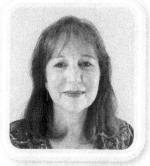

A retired teacher and speech-language pathologist, Mary Wrobel has worked with students with autism for more than thirty years and continues to consult and give workshops. She has trained both parents and professionals about puberty, and its accompanying safety, cleanliness, and health issues, as well as many other topics related to autism. This is Mary's fourth publication with Future Horizons. Her first book, *Taking Care of Myself*, won the ASA Outstanding Literary Work of the Year Award-Educational Division, as well as the iParenting Media Award. *Taking Care of Myself 2* was written for teenagers and young adults and won an iParenting Media Award. She also wrote *Autism and Girls* (co-author).

CPSIA information can be obtained
at www.ICGtesting.com
Printed in the USA
JSHW040435240523
42172JS00004B/7

9 781957 984087